the
live-longer
diet

Sally Beare

the live-longer diet

secrets of the world's longest-living people

PIATKUS

Copyright © 2003 by Sally Beare

First published in 2003 by
Judy Piatkus (Publishers) Limited
5 Windmill Street
London W1T 2JA
e-mail: info@piatkus.co.uk

The moral right of the author has been asserted

A catalogue record for this book is available from the British Library

ISBN 0 7499 2456 X

Edited by Krystyna Mayer
Text design by Paul Saunders

This book has been printed on paper manufactured
with respect for the environment using wood from
managed sustainable resources

Data manipulation by Phoenix Photosetting, Chatham, Kent
Printed and bound in Great Britain by Bookmarque Ltd, Croydon, Surrey

Contents

Part III Putting it all together   251

Acknowledgements

Thanks to:
Penny Phillips; Krystyna Mayer; Gill Bailey and Alison Sturgeon at Piatkus; Luigi Bonomi at Sheil Land; Alix Wiseman for all her help; and my husband, Khurram

Many thanks also to the following for their invaluable help with each of the places in Part 1:

Okinawa
Tariq Wasir Khan, Yumi Kashiba, Dr Akihiri Yomo
Dr Hiroto and Junko Miyagi (for their recipes)
Kagumi Yamagami and Masa Yamagami (for interviews)

Symi
Chrisa Karagianni
Irene Petridi (for interviews)
Fottini Attiti (for her recipes)
Georgios Papadopoulos

Campodimele
Paola Masi
Giuseppina Grossi (for all her invaluable help)

Marino Pecchia (for his advice and recipes)
Dr Pietro Cugini

Hunza
Jalal Haider Khan, Air Commodore Naunehal Shah, Dr Salman
Nusrat Shah, Arifa Shah, Muhammed Dost Khan, Qudsia Shah
(for their recipes)

Bama
Ji Yang, Yuan Ye

Extract from *The Pursuit of Love* by Nancy Mitford reprinted by
permission of Peters Fraser and Dunlop on behalf of: The Estate
of Nancy Mitford © 1945.

Quotation from *Stiff Upper Lip, Jeeves* by P.G. Wodehouse
published by Hutchinson, reprinted by permission of The
Random House Group Ltd.

John Steinbeck quoted by permission of Curtis Brown Group
Ltd., London.

Quotation by A. Whitney Brown printed by permission of
A. Whitney Brown.

Extract from *Conversations with God* by Neale Donald Walsch
reproduced by permission of Hodder and Stoughton Limited.

Quotation by Red Skelton printed by permission of the Estate
of Red Skelton, USA.

Preface

Why I wrote this book

Five years ago I was sitting chatting in the back of my friend's car as she negotiated a tight parking spot. Glancing in the rear-view mirror, she commented on the whiteness of my tongue. It was true – my tongue had been growing an increasingly thick white shag-pile carpet over the last two years or so. Three different GPs had been unable to offer any advice other than to take some aspirin and come back when I had a more concrete illness, and I had started talking out of the corner of my mouth in public.

After the parallel-parking incident, I knew it was time to do something. My friend suggested that I visit a nutritionist and I duly made an appointment. The woman who opened the door to me radiated vibrant good health, energy and mental well-being, and she bounded up the stairs before me. I explained to her that not only did I have this luxuriant fur on my tongue, but I also sneezed about twenty times a day, had a pain somewhere down near my appendix, frequently had a bloated, uncomfortable stomach, seemed to catch one cold after another and felt so lethargic that it was often hard to get out of bed in the morning

The nutritionist told me that all of my symptoms were related to a malfunctioning digestive system. She said that I needed to radically overhaul my diet, which was based mainly on pasta, sandwiches, wine and token salads. She didn't tell me what I couldn't eat – she just gave me a list of what I *could* eat, which included all kinds of delicious fruits and vegetables that I didn't normally bother with (avocados, asparagus, fennel and papaya, for example); pulses and wheat-free whole grains. I set off for the supermarket with my mouth watering.

Within a couple of months I was bouncing out of bed in the mornings, the pains had gone, the sneezing had stopped, I hadn't had a cold, my mood was better and my tongue was getting steadily pinker. I had also shed several pounds despite enjoying my food more than ever and eating plenty of it. Friends were full of superlatives about the dramatically different 'before' and 'after' me, and started asking me for dietary advice. I began reading about nutrition, and found that the books often contained testimonies of amazing recoveries from 'incurable' illnesses through simple changes in diet.

At about this time I had started work developing a television series about the process of ageing and some of the most cutting-edge work being done in this field. As I ate my salads of brown rice and lightly steamed mange tout seasoned with garlic and soy sauce, I read about how the huge US biotech companies are eternally searching for expensive, complicated cures for ageing and the diseases that accompany it. Meanwhile, it appeared, certain isolated pockets of people are already enjoying superb health and long life, in a way that the biotech companies can only dream of, simply because of their dietary and lifestyle habits.

Soon afterwards I gave up my television career and began training as a clinical nutritionist at the British College of Nutrition and Health. Inspired by my findings on ageing, I also started to write this book. I hope you will derive as much pleasure and satisfaction from the 'secrets' described in it as I have.

Introduction

If I had known I was going to live so long, I'd have taken better care of myself.

EUBIE BLAKE, *celebrated ragtime pianist, 1883–1983*

SCIENTISTS NOW AGREE that we could be living to around 120 years if we achieved our maximum potential lifespans. However, living to 120 does not just mean that we could be around to meet our great-grandchildren and even our great-great grandchildren. It also means that we can feel and look thirty years old at forty, eighty years old at a hundred and, most importantly, have more energy whatever age we are. In short, we can stay younger for longer. The best news is that it is never too late to start. Even those who are tired, ill and getting on in years can become biologically younger, reverse the damage, keep disease away and add years, if not decades, to their lives.

So what are the 'secrets' of living long and staying young? Ancient wisdom, thousands of authoritative studies, and recent ground-breaking research all indicate that the answer lies, above all, in what we eat. We already know that by eating the right food we can avoid some of the major killers, such as cancer and heart disease. The US Surgeon-General recently said that of the 2.2 million deaths in America each year, 1.8 million are diet-related. Now, gerontologists have also discovered that we can actually slow down or even reverse the ageing process, appear and feel younger, and prevent most ageing-related diseases with the right diet, together with certain other lifestyle habits such as taking regular exercise and avoiding stress.

It is amazing how reluctant some people are to accept these simple truths, especially when it is so much easier to eat well and take a little exercise than to find another way to slow down ageing. People have been trying, unsuccessfully, to find an instant, magical 'cure' for ageing since mankind has existed. Ancient myths derived from the Bible tell of a heavily armed archangel guarding a tree in the Garden of Eden – the Tree of Life – holding just such a cure. More recently, in the 1930s, Russian physician Professor Serge Voronoff promised wealthy patients he could reverse ageing by grafting thin slices of monkey testicle onto the insides of the scrotum, sewn together with silk stitches. There are no records of any of his patients living forever as a result, but some of them got VD, while Voronoff himself earned enough to live in immense luxury on the entire first floor of one of Paris's most expensive hotels.

Today, the pharmaceuticals companies are hopefully pumping millions of pounds into the search for an ageing cure. None of their methods, which include injecting human brains with stem cells, developing 'miracle' drugs and trying to isolate the 'gene for ageing', has yet been proven to work. Isolating the gene for ageing seems a particularly simplistic approach, since studies show that genetic inheritance is influenced by environmental factors anyway.[1] As the great scientist Ernst Krebs, Jr.

said, 'There isn't any chemical or drug that medical science could suggest that would make us healthier or better adjusted or wiser or give us hope for a longer life. There isn't a single drug or molecule in nature that can accomplish this unless that molecule exists in normal food.'[2]

Say no to the 'Tithonus option'

Living long does not have to mean existing in a world full of decrepit, senile people suffering from all sorts of age-related conditions. We do not want to be like the immortal Struldbruggs in Swift's novel *Gulliver's Travels*, who kept on growing older, iller and more miserable, and acquired 'an additional Ghastliness in Proportion to their Number of Years'. Nor would we want to go the same way as the unfortunate Greek mortal Tithonus, who was granted eternal life on the request of his goddess lover Eos. Unfortunately, Eos forgot to ask for eternal youth, and she eventually had to shut her increasingly frail, senile boyfriend in a room to gibber and babble away out of sight for eternity until, out of pity, she turned him into a grasshopper.

Unlike Tithonus and the Struldbruggs, if we look after ourselves properly we can enjoy not just improved lifespan but also improved healthspan. This is important, because in developed countries such as the UK, US and Australia, more and more people are living increasingly long lives, a phenomenon known as the 'greying' of the world's population. When the Queen first came to the throne, she sent under 300 birthday telegrams to centenarians each year. The figure is now 3,000, which is only partly accounted for by a larger population. There is a real danger that we are running out of younger generations to provide for the older people, with 11 million pensioners currently living in the UK, a figure projected to rise to 16 million by 2050. The UK government has even decided to scrap retirement at age sixty-five to help deal with the coming crisis. If we are going to be active members of the community from the age of sixty-five onwards, then it is important that we hold onto our health, and our marbles, after that age.

Living long in itself does not have to be the ultimate goal. There is no point in living to 120 if the last twenty or thirty years are spent in a nursing home, staggering about on a stick with a broken hip, forgetting what we came into the room for, and swallowing handfuls of drugs with every meal. The value of knowing that we are born with a 'bank balance' of 120 years within us is that, if we use it up slowly, we can be more active, healthier, and happier whether we are children, thirty-somethings or eighty, regardless of when we actually die.

The world's longevity hotspots

In certain parts of the world, there are people who have been proving all along that most of us are getting ill and ageing unnecessarily fast, mainly because of what we are eating, but also due to some other aspects of our lifestyles. These longevity hotspots have extraordinarily good health records and unusually high numbers of sprightly, independent nonagenarians, centenarians and super-centenarians. In Okinawa, Japan, for example, there are 34 centenarians per 100,000 people, which compares with 5 per 100,000 in the UK. Those in middle or old age behave and look like much younger people, and illness – *any* kind of illness, from headaches to cancer – is rare.

We know that it is environmental factors rather than good genes that are primarily responsible for the health and youth of these people, because studies show that when they move to other countries and adopt local diets they also develop local diseases and other signs of ageing. The existence of such people also disproves the argument that the only reason for our current high rates of degenerative disease, such as heart disease and cancer, is that we are living longer.

The five longevity hot spots discussed in this book are:

- *Okinawa*, an island in Japan.

- *Campodimele*, a village in Southern Italy.

- *Symi*, an island in Greece.

- *Hunza*, a valley in north-west Pakistan.

- *Bama*, a county in southern China.

The 'secrets' of longevity

This book reveals the 'secrets' behind these populations' exceptional good health and longevity. In fact, there are really no secrets at all: common sense and some diet and lifestyle habits are all there is to it. Delicious fresh, locally grown and caught foods, an active lifestyle, plenty of fresh air and a positive approach to life's challenges are the factors that give these people their edge. With some extra effort, most of these elements can be incorporated into the lives of the rest of us. True, you cannot buy fresh air or a happy marriage in a supermarket, but anyone can find ways to reduce stress, take more exercise and look after themselves if they really want to. As for the food, the ingredients for all of the recipes in this book and more like them are available from supermarkets and health-food shops.

Enjoying food

The dishes of the people in the five longevity hot spots are not only nutritious but also delicious. The rule is to obtain good-quality, fresh ingredients and then to interfere with them as little as possible so that the flavours are allowed to come through. People complain about 'health food' being bland, but health food does not have to mean just a piece of apple and a rice cake. It can and should mean dishes of fresh new vegetables and herbs, pulses or fish, infused with the flavour of garlic and onions, ginger and soy sauce, a little red wine or any other of the hundreds of ingredients involved in healthy cooking. The principles of a healthy diet are simple: plenty of fresh fruits and vegetables, whole grains rather than refined foods, the right kinds of oils, not too much meat and short cooking times.

We don't want to be eating a diet devised in a laboratory and tested on rats. We want usable, delicious recipes perfected over generations, not simply because they give us health, but also because they taste good. In Part I, I have included examples of the types of recipe prepared by the five populations I discuss in this book. These recipes – and others like them – will help you to forget about calories and willpower, and to serve the kind of food that you and your friends will love and appreciate. They will also help you to achieve optimum levels of energy and health each day and to feel younger for longer. Hippocrates, the ancient Greek 'Father of Medicine', was said to have uttered these famous words: 'Let food be your medicine and medicine be your food.' The good news is that food doesn't have to taste like medicine for this to be true.

Why this book applies to you

In order to stave off degenerative diseases and enjoy optimum health, we have to get the full range of nutrients. These include at least seventeen to twenty minerals, thirteen vitamins, eleven essential amino acids and two essential fatty acids ('essential' meaning that they are essential for health and that they cannot be made in the body). At the absolute minimum, we should eat at least five portions of fresh fruits and vegetables each day, and preferably ten. Yet most Western diets include far less than this, and the UK Food Standards Agency found that only 36 per cent of people in the UK are even aware of the recommendation.

We are made of food, and what we eat affects our minds, bodies and spirits. Obesity is on the rise in developed countries, yet, increasingly, many people are starving to death – that is, they are starved of nutrients. Calorie-rich foods, such as pastries and sugary snacks, add the pounds but take out the things our bodies need to be healthy, such as vitamins and minerals. In tandem with this, degenerative disease is on the rise. In 1988, the US Surgeon-General's Report on Health and Nutrition concluded that almost 75 per cent of deaths in the United States involve nutritional deficiency. On the whole, specific illnesses cannot be cured by specific remedies or drugs. Most illnesses, and accelerated ageing, are caused by one basic factor – a diet deficient in nutrients and excessive in toxins.

Too many of us are resigned to feeling lethargic, getting regular headaches, suffering from PMS, having mood swings and sugar cravings, and developing degenerative diseases as we age. Ulcers, indigestion and allergies are all, quite wrongly, accepted as inevitable burdens of living and growing old. Anyone who has suffered from any of these and is sceptical about the immense power of diet to affect well-being has not tried eating truly healthily. The benefits commonly experienced by those on a high-nutrient diet include better skin, weight loss, increased energy, the disappearance of minor ailments, an ability to jump out of bed in the mornings, improved libido and a reduced risk of long-term illness. If, on top of that, we can live an extra ten or twenty years of quality life, surely it is worth a try.

The top killer illnesses are preventable

You have no need to fear the top killer illnesses in the UK (these are also common killers in other societies in the developed world, such as the US, Australia and white South Africa). With the exception of ageing (which can be slowed down considerably), they are all largely preventable.

Ageing

Until scientists find a way to make us immortal, ageing and death will be inescapable facts of life. In the 1960s Dr Leonard Hayflick discovered that the ten million, million cells in the human body are only capable of dividing a certain number of times before they start to look old, reach their limit and die out. This phenomenon, known as the Hayflick Limit, shows that we are born with a kind of 'ageing clock' within us, which gives us a certain maximum allotted amount of time on Earth (now known to be about 120 years).

The most common causes of death in the UK today unfortunately do not include getting to the end of our Hayflick Limit – nearly all of us die while our cells are still dividing, as a result of disease or accelerated ageing. In the UK, the average man can expect to live to 75.1, and the average woman to 79.9, potentially depriving us of an extra 40 years. Yet not only can we slow the ageing process, but we can also undo damage already done. Renowned gerontologist and nutrition expert John McDougall writes: 'Every day I see broken bodies transformed into more radiant, active, agile, brighter people. The secret for successful ageing is almost too simple to believe – it is a healthy diet, moderate exercise, and clean habits. But the results are no less than a miracle.'[3]

Cardiovascular disease

CVD, or disease of the heart and blood vessels, is the number one cause of death in the UK (around 300,000 people die annually from coronary heart disease, or CHD, and stroke in the UK), as well as in the US, Australia and South Africa. It is also one of the most preventable diseases there is. Leading US nutritionist Dr Michael Colgan says, 'Do not fear cardiovascular disease. It's the easiest of all man-made diseases to prevent and even to reverse, if only you follow the right nutrition, plus a little easy exercise to blow away the cobwebs.'[4] By reducing your risk of heart attack, you also slash the risk of getting diabetes, which is closely linked.

'Couch potato syndrome', obesity, smoking and poor diet have been blamed in countless studies for the high rates of heart disease in the West. Forty-five per cent of the South African population is classified as obese, while the British Heart Foundation states that 'One reason why CHD rates are high in the UK is because the average diet is so unhealthy. In particular fat intake – especially of saturated fat – in the UK is too high, and fruit and vegetable consumption is too low.'[5] By contrast, the long-lived people that are described in this book frequently reach their nineties and hundreds, yet medical researchers have found that they have extremely low rates of heart disease and exceptionally youthful arteries.

Cancer

Cancer is now overtaking heart disease as the leading cause of death in the UK, killing approximately 150,000 people annually.[6] Cancer rates are also among the top causes of death in the US, Australia and South Africa. Yet cancer is highly avoidable. Three of the most common cancers in these countries – breast, prostate and bowel cancers – are all strongly linked with diet and lifestyle habits. Even the ultra-conservative American Cancer Society has said that 90 per cent of colorectal cancer cases are preventable.[7] Cancer expert Dr Patrick Quillan says in his book *Beating Cancer with Nutrition*: 'The body is equipped to deal with cancer. . . but this process relies heavily on nutrition . . . Proper nutrition could prevent 50–90% of all cancer.'

As far as cancer treatments go, chemotherapy might have its place, but it has unpleasant side effects and only works to a limited extent (one in three people in the UK gets cancer and one in four dies of it, so you don't need to be a genius at maths to work out that chemotherapy isn't a miracle cure). However, there are effective alternative treatments available whose only side effects are good ones. The famous cancer therapist Dr Max Gerson, for example, claimed a 30 per cent success rate for *terminal* cancers alone for his nutritional therapy. Another treatment using vitamin B17 (or Laetrile) has been found in experiments to have an *82 per cent response rate*. Vitamin B17 is found in apricot kernels, which are eaten in large quantities by the cancer-free Hunzakuts. To read more about the fascinating story behind the vitamin B17 treatment and its suppression by the pharmaceuticals industry, see Phillip Day's *Cancer: Why*

We're Still Dying To Know the Truth.[8] The Gerson Therapy and vitamin B17 treatments are practised in some cancer therapy centres – see Useful Addresses (*page 284*) for details.

Respiratory disease

This is the third leading cause of death in the UK, with diseases such as lung cancer and pneumonia killing around 90,000 people annually. Lung cancer is mainly caused by smoking while pneumonia tends to strike at the very old and frail; many cases of pneumonia are also caught in hospital (*see below*).

The National Health Service

Around 41,650 people are killed each year as a result of blunders in the UK's National Health Service. This astounding figure – the equivalent of 130 jumbo jet crashes annually – is part of a wider total figure of 850,000 'adverse events', according to a 2001 study by the Chief Medical Officer.[9] This makes the NHS easily the fourth biggest cause of premature death. It is not just the NHS system that is to blame, but medicine itself – in the US, 'death from doctoring' is the third leading cause of death. Most of these deaths are caused by adverse reactions to the wrong types or dosages of pharmaceutical drugs, with 21,353 reports of such reactions in the UK in 2001, according to the Medicines Control Agency. Other incidents causing premature death involve unnecessary surgery, infections caught in hospitals, equipment failure and other errors, including absurd lapses of care like being trapped by bedrails and mattresses, leading to asphyxiation.

Doctors and modern medicine are an essential part of our healthcare system, at least when functioning properly, as anyone who has been in a car accident or had any other life-threatening condition requiring immediate surgery will testify. However, drugs and surgery are not always the best solutions for chronic degenerative illnesses such as cancer, heart conditions or digestive diseases. Preventive medicine is best – according to the *New England Journal of Medicine*, '90 per cent of patients who visit doctors have conditions that will either improve on their own or are out of reach of modern medicine's ability to solve.'[10]

Digestive disorders

These kill approximately 20,000 people in the UK annually. It goes without saying that digestive problems are directly linked to diet. By following the advice in this book you should be able to have a wonderful working digestion with all the health benefits it brings with it.

I

The world's five longevity hotspots

This section describes the five most remarkable pockets of long-lived populations in the world, where the people are bursting with health, live for record-breaking numbers of years, and are active and vigorous even past a hundred years of age. It discusses the basic reasons for their remarkable longevity and provides sample recipes illustrating the types of food that they eat. Part II explains the 'secrets' behind these people's longevity in more detail and offers suggestions that will enable you to apply them to your life.

Okinawa, island of world-record longevity

•

THE OKINAWAN ARCHIPELAGO, a group of 161 coral islands in the East China Sea, is home to the people who, out of everyone in the world, can truly claim to possess the elixir of lasting youth. In this verdant, bountiful 'Galapagos of the East', the people have beautiful skins, lustrous dark hair and slim, agile bodies long past middle age. The main diseases of the West are at the lowest levels in the world, suicide is almost unheard of and the word 'retirement' does not exist in the local dialect.

Okinawa's centenarians and super-centenarians do not spend their last years in nursing homes but enjoy full, active lives right to the end. One local celebrity is a ninety-seven-year-old karate teacher, famous for recently defeating an ex-boxing champion in his thirties. When Okinawans do die, they die quickly, often without any known illness. With 34 centenarians per 100,000 (compared with 5 per 100,000 in the UK), and an unusually high number of people aged over 105, Okinawans are officially the longest lived people on the planet.

Heart disease, stroke and cancer, so common in the West, are at the lowest levels in the world in Okinawa, and are only 60 per cent of that of the rest of Japan, which itself has unusually low levels. Okinawans have 80 per cent fewer heart attacks than Americans, and examinations by doctors have revealed unusually young arteries and low cholesterol levels. Breast cancer is so rare that mammographies are not needed, and most older men have not even heard of prostate cancer. Overall, there is 40 per cent less cancer in Okinawa than there is in the West; and when Okinawans do get cancer they are over twice as likely to survive it.

Since 1975, a group of distinguished doctors has been studying the extraordinary health and longevity of the Okinawans, including 400 centenarians and super-centenarians; their results have been published in their recent book, *The Okinawa Way*.[1] The Centenarian Study researchers found that Okinawans are generally in 'outstanding health'.

The first person authors Dr Bradley Willcox and Dr Craig Willcox examined was a 100-year-old man, whom they first took to be about seventy, and of whom they found that 'after a hundred years of use, there was basically nothing wrong with his body'. The doctors found that even in old age, Okinawans have youthful immune systems, very low rates of osteoporosis, fit, attractive bodies, high levels of sex hormones and excellent mental health.

The authors of the study conclude in their book that the 'secrets' of these people are almost all replicable in the West, and are primarily to do with diet, as well as some other lifestyle factors such as regular exercise and a positive mental outlook. Unfortunately, the younger generations of Okinawans are abandoning the traditional diet and turning to the fast-food joints that surround the American air bases on the islands. Their rates of 'Western' diseases such as heart attack and cancer are going up accordingly, illustrating that genes only have a minor role to play in their longevity.

An exemplary diet

The traditional Okinawan diet follows all the main rules of healthy, balanced eating, and as you will see in this book, it is just the kind of diet to promote good health and long life. The Okinawans have a saying, *Ishoku-dogen*, meaning, literally, 'food and medicine from the same source'. Their food is rich in anti-cancer, anti-ageing antioxidants – the miracle molecules that neutralise ageing free radicals (*see page 123* for full explanation). The traditional diet is based mainly on sweet potatoes, leafy greens and whole grains, and supplemented with fish, rice, pork and soya products. Okinawan cuisine is unique to Japan in that it is influenced by both Chinese and Japanese cooking; with its pork and vegetable dishes from China and fish and seaweed dishes from Japan, the diet contains a wide range of nutrients. Only minimal amounts of age-promoting fat, meat, sugar, refined carbohydrates and stimulants are consumed.

As is the case with all long-lived populations, the Okinawans also benefit from a low-calorie diet. They eat plenty in terms of volume – in fact, the Centenarian Study researchers found that they actually eat more food by weight than North Americans – but they only eat around 1,500 calories daily, which is about 40 per cent fewer calories than the average North American. Okinawans do not go hungry because their high-vegetable diet is rich in nutrients and bulky fibre. Japanese people also tend to be of slighter build than the average Westerner, and therefore need fewer calories – 1,500 is probably too low for Westerners. The Japanese, including Okinawans, have a saying, *hara hachi bu*, meaning 'only eat until you are only eight parts full'.

Eating exactly what you need and no more, as the Okinawans do, has been shown by longevity scientists to be the only proven method of extending human lifespan, and this type of eating is thought to be one of the main reasons for their longevity (Chapter 6 explains the dramatic effects of a low-calorie, nutrient-dense diet).[2] It is thought that the reason why this type of diet extends lifespan is that it keeps down levels of free radicals, which are now known to be the number one culprits behind accelerated ageing and degenerative disease (see Chapter 7 for more about free radicals). The Centenarian Study researchers found that Okinawans do indeed have wonderfully low blood levels of free radicals, with hundred-year-olds measuring just over half the level of the free radical, lipid peroxide, of the average 'normal' seventy-year-old.[3]

The importance of fresh vegetables

Over a third of the average Okinawan meal consists of fresh organic vegetables, packed with free-radical-quenching anti-oxidants and fibre. (Chapter 7 explains more about fruits and vegetables and why they are a crucial part of longevity eating.) Okinawans grow their own organic vegetables all the year round on nutrient-rich soil, and in Kijoka village, home to the longest lived islanders, the soil has been left particularly rich in minerals by the sea which covered it 150 years ago.

Government anti-cancer recommendations in the UK and the US are to eat five or more servings of fruits and vegetables daily. The Okinawans eat around six servings of vegetables and one of fruits. They like to make their food look appetising and by employing several differently coloured foods in their meals – for example orange sweet potatoes and green leafy vegetables

– they receive the benefits of a range of antioxidants working together, as well as galvanising their digestive juices into action.

Vegetable peel, full of extra flavour and antioxidants – the two go together – is kept or even used separately to make vegetable peel dishes, such as radish peel salad. The most common way to prepare vegetables is by gently stir-frying them for a short amount of time, so that minimal nutrients are lost. Stir-fries nearly always start with antioxidant-rich onions, and frying is done in canola oil, which is a healthier option than other vegetable oils (apart from olive oil – see Chapter 11). Popular vegetables include carrots, cabbage, watercress, white radish and oriental greens (similar to spinach or pak choi).

Sweet potatoes have been a staple of the Okinawan diet ever since they were introduced in the seventeenth century; they are so important that there is even an old Okinawan greeting, *nmu kamatooin*, meaning 'Are you getting enough sweet potato?' Sweet potatoes, as their vivid orange flesh shows, are rich in the anti-cancer antioxidant beta-carotene, as well as in calcium, magnesium, potassium, folic acid, vitamin C, vitamin E and lycopene. They are also low on the glycaemic index (therefore good for blood sugar levels), and high in fibre. (Chapter 12 contains more on the glycaemic index and blood sugar levels.)

Goya, a bitter, marrow-like vegetable resembling a cactus, is a mainstay of the diet, eaten practically every day and for cele-bratory meals. Along with other ingredients, it is usually put in a stir-fry called *goya champuru* (*champuru* meaning 'mixed'). Goya is used as a folk remedy for various ailments, is said to be a male aphrodisiac and contains high levels of vitamin C, even when cooked. Goya is available in the West in oriental super-markets; alternatively, you can use courgettes, marrow or squash.

Seaweed

Antioxidant-rich seaweed is used to flavour dishes and make stocks. It is very dense in nutrients, so only small quantities are needed. As well as antioxidants, seaweed contains essential fatty acids – the fats that are an essential part of our diet (*see page 163*) – and is a good source of protein and crucial minerals such as calcium, magnesium, zinc and iodine. According to the Japanese, seaweed prevents grey hair and baldness, which is why it is added to Japanese hair products. Popular types of seaweed are kombu, nori, hijiki and wakame, all of which are available in oriental and health-food shops in the West.

Fruits

Okinawans eat at least one portion of fruit each day, as part of their seven daily servings of nutrient-rich fruits and vegetables. Since vegetables contain higher levels of nutrients than fruits, this is a perfectly good ratio. Some of the fruits most commonly eaten are papayas, watermelons, bananas, pineapples and tangerines. Fruits are eaten raw, and so provides beneficial digestive enzymes – papaya and pineapple contain the enzymes papain and bromelain respectively (if you have problems with constipation, try eating one of these fruits and you will see for yourself how useful they are).

Fish

Okinawans are fishermen as well as farmers, and regularly – around two or three times a week – eat fish caught fresh from clean seas. Oily fish such as tuna, mackerel and salmon contain the omega 3 essential fatty acids (EFAs) which build our brains and nervous systems, are vital for the health of every cell in our bodies, and are thought to protect against cancer, heart disease, inflammatory disease, dry skin and hair, PMS, mental illness and practically any other ailment you care to mention.

Fish is also a complete protein while being far more digestible than meat and much lower in saturated fats. EFAs additionally aid metabolism, so that despite being fats, they can help you lose weight. It is no coincidence that all of the long-lived populations described in this book get their daily EFAs (see Chapters 11 and 16 for more about why you must get these fats in your diet, particularly if you are pregnant or breast-feeding).

It is a shame that fish, especially farmed fish such as salmon, can contain high levels of toxins such as PCBs (polychlorinated biphenyls), growth enhancers and pesticides. The UK Food Standards Agency maintains that the benefits of eating one or two portions of oily fish weekly outweigh the dangers; try to buy organic or wild fish if you can. Mackerel, sardines and herring are less likely to be polluted than salmon, and tuna should be limited as it can contain high levels of mercury. You can also get fish-oil capsules – make sure you use a good brand.

Soya

Soya is a superfood, revered the world over by nutrition experts and credited for the low levels of breast and prostate cancer in Asian soya-eating populations. It is also an Okinawan favourite – the islanders eat around three ounces of soya daily, mainly in the form of miso and tofu, and also as soy sauce, tempeh and soya milk. Studies indicate that soya protects against hormonal cancers (such as breast and prostate cancer) with its plant oestrogens, called phytoestrogens, which balance hormone levels.[4] People who eat soya regularly also have less PMS and hormone-related problems such as polycystic ovaries.[5]

Soya protects the heart and blood vessels in several ways. It contains antioxidants that protect blood vessels by preventing the oxidation of 'bad' LDL cholesterol; it also lowers LDL cholesterol levels.[6] (See Chapter 10 for more on cholesterol.) Research has shown that the isoflavones in soya strengthen blood vessels and inhibit the development of atherosclerosis.[7] Soya contains omega 3 and omega 6 EFAs and blood-thinning vitamin E. Soya is also partly credited for the low incidence of hip fractures in Okinawa and other soya-eating areas, as it contains both calcium and magnesium.[8] It is an excellent source of protein, as it contains all eight essential amino acids. (See Chapter 9 for more about the advantages of vegetable protein.)

Soya occasionally gets some bad press. Studies have shown that soya beans have some toxic properties and may be harmful when eaten in large amounts. However, these findings were based on tests in which rats were given large amounts of soya and little or nothing else, whereas Okinawans eat moderate amounts *as part of a nutrient-rich, well-balanced diet*. One recent study found that Japanese men in Hawaii who ate two or more servings of tofu per week experienced more brain ageing than those who did not.[9] Clearly, despite its benefits, soya is not a perfect food, and it should be remembered that with soya, as with all longevity foods, moderation and an overall well-balanced diet is the key.

Whole grains and noodles

Around six to seven servings of grains, mainly whole grains, are eaten every day by Okinawans, making up about a third of their diet. About three of these servings consist of white rice, which has started to replace the traditional sweet potato. This is just about the only area of the Okinawan diet that could do with improvement, as brown rice is better for digestion than white rice, and contains more nutrients.

The other three servings consist of wheat udon noodles or delicious grey soba noodles made from buckwheat. Buckwheat has been thought of as a health food in Japan for thousands of years. It contains anti-cancer vitamin B17, and is also very effective in reducing high blood pressure as it contains capillary-strengthening rutin. Chapter 4 on Hunza contains more about the incredible properties of vitamin B17.

Another heart-friendly property of buckwheat is its high fibre content, which helps remove excess cholesterol from the body. Buckwheat helps the liver deal with excess alcohol, which is why soba noodle soup and soba water is served to hungover businessmen in soba shops in Japan. Whole grains such as buckwheat also help to regulate blood sugar levels, which slows down ageing. Chapter 12 explains why you should include whole grains rather than refined carbohydrates in your diet.

Lean meat used sparingly

Okinawans love pork and they have it with many of their dishes. However, although meat is becoming increasingly common in the Okinawan diet (especially since the Americans introduced spam after World War II), traditionally meat such as pork and goat were eaten only a few times a year or used in small amounts to flavour vegetable-based dishes.

Meat eaten by the Okinawans has the fat trimmed off it and is then usually boiled to make stock, which makes it comparatively lean and digestible. The Okinawans only derive 24 per cent of their calories from fat, which is well under the Western dietary recommendations of 30 per cent of calories; in addition, only a small amount of these calories comes from unhealthy saturated fats (see Chapter 11). All of the long-lived people described in this book eat similarly limited amounts of meat; Chapter 9 explains why this is such an important factor in any longevity diet.

Low salt consumption

Like the other populations discussed here, the Okinawans use salt very sparingly in their cooking. They therefore do not suffer from illnesses related to high salt consumption, such as high blood pressure. In addition, Okinawans do not have the relatively high incidence of stomach cancer suffered by mainland Japanese, which has been attributed by the Centenarian Study researchers to their low consumption of salt. Salt encourages infection from the virus *Helicobacter pylori*, which is linked to stomach cancer and stomach ulcers.

Traditionally, Okinawans had to extract salt from sea water for home consumption, so they only ate small amounts; in addition, sea salt has the benefit of being rich in magnesium, which counteracts the blood-pressure-raising effects of salt. Instead of flavouring their broths with salt, Okinawans use dashi, a stock made from seaweed and dried fish (*see page 30* for recipe).

Fermented rice wine

Awamori is the Okinawan equivalent of sake, a fermented rice wine used for cooking and seasoning as well as for drinking (*see page 33* for recipe). Awamori and sake contain polyphenols that prevent hardening of the arteries and seem to protect certain brain functions against the ageing process: recent studies from the National Institute for Longevity in Tokyo have shown that middle-aged and older people who drink moderate amounts of wine or sake actually have higher intelligence quotients than teetotallers.[10]

Beware the law of diminishing returns, however, since a high intake of more than two drinks daily is associated with liver damage and an increased risk of certain cancers. One recent study has shown that drinking just one glass of wine daily increases a woman's chances of getting breast cancer by about 6 per cent, as it increases oestrogen levels.[11] Okinawan women, however, enjoy around one drink a day, and they have exceptionally low rates of breast cancer, so other factors (such as high soya intake) should be taken into account.

Jasmine green tea and calcium-rich water

Okinawans drink about three cups a day of delicious green tea scented with jasmine flowers. Green tea contains more antioxidants than any other food or drink, as well as catechins, which stop cancer cells from reproducing. Green tea has been found to protect against cancers of the oesophagus, colon, breast, lung, stomach and skin.[12] It is thought that one of the reasons why mainland Japanese have lower levels of lung cancer than they should, considering the amount they smoke, is because they drink around six cups of green tea daily. Black tea is not as beneficial to health as green tea as it contains more caffeine, but studies show that both black tea and green tea reduce heart disease and stroke by blocking the build-up of plaque and lowering blood cholesterol.[13]

Okinawans have also traditionally drunk plenty of calcium-rich local water; the calcium helps to prevent osteoporosis and keeps the body slightly alkaline, which is how it needs to be for optimum health.

Medicinal plants

Around 460 varieties of herb are grown in Okinawa. They are used for medicinal purposes as well as for flavouring foods.

- Turmeric, which is used to enhance soups and fish and chicken dishes, contains the antioxidant curcumin, which has been found in tests to boost the immune system, aid digestion, reduce inflammation, prevent blood clotting and help the liver to detoxify.

- The herb mugwort, commonly drunk in tea or awamori, is thought to reduce a range of problems, particularly respiratory illnesses such as tuberculosis and the common cold.

- Shiitake mushrooms are used as a folk medicine in Okinawa and are becoming an area of important research in the West because of their effective immune-system-boosting properties.

- Ginger, used in many local dishes, has anti-viral properties and helps alleviate morning sickness and nausea.

Regular physical exercise

Again in common with all five of the long-lived populations discussed in this book, traditional Okinawans get plenty of exercise and fresh air every day, since most of them are fishermen or farmers; they continue to work hard outdoors even into their eighties. They also make a point of taking regular aerobic exercise, including martial arts and traditional dance, as well as engaging in gardening and walking. They enjoy weekly matches of gateball, a game similar to bowling, which local doctors say keeps them out in the sunshine and allows them to vent stress. Okinawans are exceptionally fit and supple; even 100-year-olds will sit cross-legged on the floor for long periods of time.

Exercise is essential for cardiovascular health as it keeps the heart muscle healthy, and it also tones the abdominal muscles that are used for peristalsis, the movement of faecal matter through the gut. Weight-bearing exercise such as walking helps to maintain bone density and is thought to be one reason why there is a low osteoporosis rate among Okinawans. Taking exercise outside also ensures that the action of sunlight on the body produces vitamin D, which is needed for bone health. Chapter 19 contains further information on why exercise is so important for good health and long life.

Brain fitness

The old and super-old Okinawans do not retire but keep busy even in their nineties or hundreds; they garden, socialise, work in the fields or maintain cottage industries making handicrafts. The old and very old are revered, not made to feel redundant as they often are in the West, and when people attain lofty ages they are dressed in red and paraded through the streets in a celebration of their achievement.

Having a sense of purpose in later life is thought by gerontologists to maintain vigour and promote longevity. Staying active after retirement has been found to have a major impact on the rate of ageing, and intricate work with the hands such as weaving fabric may stimulate the brain to keep it fresh. Chapter 20 contains advice on how you can use your brain to stay young.

Low stress

High stress levels are thought to speed up the ageing process and cause disease, so it is not surprising that the Okinawans have exceptionally low stress levels. People live at a relaxed pace, known locally as 'Okinawa Time', and generally turn up late for everything. You do not see urgent or worried faces in Okinawa; instead people sing as they walk through the streets or when they are working in the fields.

It is not as if there were no external stressors in Okinawa – the islanders suffered much poverty and loss during World War II, and they also experience death and some divorce. However, the Centenarian Study researchers found that Okinawans have a great deal of self-confidence and 'unyieldingness', which help them to cope well with life's crises. Okinawans regularly practise meditation, which studies suggest can significantly slow the ageing process.[14] They also have strong spiritual beliefs, sharing their problems with gods and ancestors. Okinawan women in particular have been found to have an enhanced sense of well-being as a result of their strong spiritual beliefs.[15]

Close-knit communities

The Okinawans have an expression, *yuimaaru*, meaning 'mutual aid and reciprocity'. Although the elderly often live on their own and enjoy a healthy sense of independence, they also receive plenty of tender loving care from friends and family, and neighbours will often leave food on each other's doorsteps if it is needed. *Yuimaaru* also embodies the idea of living in harmony with nature and the idea of symbiosis with people and the environment.

According to the Centenarian Study researchers, *yuimaaru* extends lifespan and protects from illness, partly by boosting the immune system. *Ichariba chode* is an expression that means to interact with everyone as though they were your own kin, so that everyone feels loved and wanted. People socialise frequently, dropping in on each other for breakfast or playing music on each other's porches in the evenings.

Kiyoko Fukuchi, 102 years old

Kiyoko Fukuchi is a typical Okinawan super-centenarian. Lively and enthusiastic for her age, she considers herself to be in good shape and has no complaints. With her smooth skin and supple body, she looks 'very young', according to those who know her, and even her eyesight is good enough for her to see without glasses. Although she lives with her daughter, she is independent and capable, doing her own chores without any help, and going for walks whenever the weather permits. She also enjoys visiting friends and family, and attends local old people's get-togethers twice a month.

Kiyoko believes that the reason why she is still in such good condition at this age is that she has always eaten well and stayed active. Her diet consists mainly of ample amounts of home-grown vegetables and locally caught fish. She also eats aloe with every meal – aloe is used in the West as an effective remedy for soothing and healing the digestive tract. She has never eaten much meat, and has never had access to junk foods or sweets.

OKINAWAN DOS AND DON'TS

Okinawans do:

- Eat a high-nutrient, low-calorie diet.
- Eat a well-balanced, varied diet.
- Eat plenty of fresh vegetables and fruits, grown organically and locally.
- Get plenty of essential fatty acids, mainly from fish.
- Eat soya regularly, which balances hormones and provides vegetable protein.
- Eat whole grains rather than refined carbohydrates.
- Drink moderate amounts of alcohol.
- Drink green tea and calcium-rich water.
- Get regular exercise.
- Remain mentally active throughout their lives.
- Have a healthy psycho-spiritual outlook and low stress.
- Live in happy, close-knit communities.

Okinawans don't:

- Overeat.
- Overcook their food.
- Eat sugar.
- Consume much salt.
- Eat refined or processed foods.
- Eat much meat or dairy foods.
- Drink tea or coffee (except for green tea).
- Drink alcohol in excess.

Okinawa Recipes

DASHI

This is a classic Japanese stock made from seaweed and dried fish flakes from the bonito fish. It is a staple of many dishes and is also used as a medicinal soup to maintain and restore vigour. Use it as a versatile base for your own invented recipes using noodles, soya and vegetables.

2 strips kombu seaweed
Approx 5 g bonito flakes (available in 3 g sachets from oriental supermarkets)
1 tbsp soy sauce

1. Boil the kombu for 3 to 4 minutes in a small pan of water (use about half a pint of water). Remove from the heat.
2. Add the bonito flakes and return to the heat. Remove from the heat just as the water returns to the boil.
3. Leave to stand for 5 minutes or until the bonito flakes sink. Strain and reserve the liquid. Discard the solids (if you are making dashi again soon you can reuse them).
4. Add the soy sauce.

PORK NOODLES WITH DASHI

This is extremely easy to make and delicious – you will be amazed by the authenticity of the flavour, which comes from the dashi. Eat it with some steamed vegetables on the side, or add a few sliced vegetables such as cabbage or broccoli after step 2.

Serves 1–2

100 g (4 oz) cooked pork slices or salmon
1 tbsp olive or canola oil
½ clove garlic
1 tbsp dashi
1–2 tbsp soy sauce (use the traditionally brewed, low-salt kind)
1 tsp sake/sweet white wine
240 ml (8 fl oz) stock (pork or vegetable if using salmon)
100 g (4 oz) oriental noodles, preferably udon noodles (buckwheat
udon noodles are available in oriental supermarkets)
3 stalks green onions, chopped very fine

1. If using pork, boil the meat in about a pint of water for 25 minutes. Skim the fat off the top of the water and keep the rest to use as stock.
2. Heat the oil in a wok or frying pan. Add the garlic and fry gently for a minute or two, without letting it brown. You can bring down the frying temperature by adding a tablespoon of stock.
3. Add the pork or salmon and stir for a few seconds.
4. Add the dashi, soy sauce, sake and stock, and bring to the boil.
5. Add the noodles and heat.
6. Garnish with the onion and serve.

SAUTÉED TOFU AND VEGETABLES

You can use any leftover vegetables for this, such as broccoli, cauliflower, green peppers or pak choi.

Serves 2
1–2 tbsp olive or canola oil
1 onion, chopped
1 clove garlic, chopped (optional)
1 tsp fresh ginger, chopped (optional)
50 g (2 oz) GM-free tofu, diced
1 carrot, sliced
100g (4oz) cabbage, sliced
100g (4oz) bean sprouts
1–2 tsp soy sauce
1 tbsp dashi (optional)

1. Heat the oil in a frying pan or work and cook the onion on a fairly high heat for a few minutes, stirring continuously until it is soft but not brown. Add the garlic and/or ginger if you are using them.
2. Add the tofu, then the carrot, then the cabbage, followed by the bean sprouts. Keep stirring for a few minutes.
3. Add a little soy sauce to taste, and/or a spoonful of dashi if you are using it. Cook for another 2 or 3 minutes, then serve.

GRILLED FISH WITH GREENS AND SWEET POTATO

There is no particular Okinawan recipe for this. When the Okinawans eat fish, they usually just grill it and eat it with vegetables and rice or sweet potato.

Serves 1
1 sweet potato
300 g (11 oz) oily fish, such as salmon, fresh tuna, mackerel or fresh
sardines
Juice of 1 lemon
Olive oil
150 g (5 oz) spinach or pak choi

1. Either bake or mash the sweet potato – if baking, put it in an oven preheated to 190° C/375° F/gas mark 5 for about 30 minutes before cooking the fish (sweet potatoes usually take around 40 minutes to cook).
2. Grill the fish with a little lemon and olive oil for 5 to 10 minutes on each side until cooked.
3. Steam the greens for a couple of minutes and serve with the rest.

PORK AND VEGETABLE SOUP WITH SAKE

Okinawans make this when someone is unwell, but it can be enjoyed any time. If pork is not available, they sometimes use fish – if you want to use fish, boil it for a much shorter period, and make sure you use really fresh fish.

Serves 4–5
300 g (11 oz) pork
300 g (11 oz) pork liver (optional)
Sake or awamori (fermented rice wine)
3 potatoes, chopped
1 carrot, chopped
1 tbsp miso (soy paste)
1–2 tsp chopped ginger
1–2 spring onions, cut into thin matchsticks

1. Cut the meat into small pieces and leave to marinate in a bowl of sake or awamori for 20 minutes.
2. Boil the meat in a pan of water (the amount you use depends on how watery you want your soup to be); skim any fat from the top of the water as it forms.
3. After 15–20 minutes, add the vegetables, then continue cooking for 10 minutes.

4. Remove from the heat and stir in the miso and chopped ginger.
5. Garnish with the spring onions and serve with a glass of warm sake.

RICE WITH SEAWEED

The Okinawans make a complicated version of this using a rice cooker; this is a quick and easy variation to be used as a side dish for fish and/or vegetables. You can use kombu seaweed and cut it into strips, or hijiki seaweed, which comes in tiny dark strips.

Serves 2
200 g (7 oz) brown rice
2 strips kombu seaweed or hijiki seaweed
1 onion, chopped small
1 clove garlic, chopped small
1 tbsp olive or canola oil
1 tsp sesame oil
1–2 tbsp soy sauce

1. Wash and cook the rice.
2. If using kombu seaweed, boil for 20 minutes, then cut into matchstick-sized slivers with scissors or a knife. If using hijiki seaweed, soak for 15 minutes in warm water, then drain.
3. Sauté the onion and garlic in the oil, add the cooked rice, then the seaweed.
4. Add a little sesame oil (if using) and the soy sauce, and stir for another minute or two.

chapter
2

Symi, home of truly ancient Greeks

•

THE FISHY MEDITERRANEAN DIET, so well known for its wonderful health benefits, is perhaps best exemplified on the Greek island of Symi. Greece is famous for the good health of its population, especially on Crete, but it is on Symi that you will find the most truly ancient Greeks. Even when they are old, Symiots are young – men in their seventies and eighties are well toned and vigorous. They flirt openly with any woman who catches their eye, which is hardly surprising, because the women on Symi are also well toned and vigorous, with beautiful skin and hair.

Right up to their nineties, both men and women can be found chasing after their herds, collecting herbs, making yoghurt and gardening. Everyone on Symi knows someone who has passed the age of 100, and a traditional birthday greeting is 'May you live to be 100 and more!' The population of Symi is small, at a mere 2,700, and the number of centenarians and ninety-year-olds varies from year to year.

However, epidemiologists have found that Symi has the best health records and highest life expectancy for the region.[1]

The rocky outcrops of Symi are softened by clear blue water full of fish, and the welcoming sea breeze is scented with pine, sage and eucalyptus. In the main village, neoclassical houses painted in blues and creams rise steeply above one another, each looking out over the harbour and the spectacular Turkish coastline a few kilometres away across the Aegean Sea.

Each morning, a flotilla of brightly painted fishing boats sets off from the harbour to get in the day's catch, returning in the evening to deliver delicacies such as squid, lobster, giant sardines and prawns to the restaurants along the harbour and the houses up above. Ropes of garlic and bunches of herbs picked from the hillside hang everywhere along the seafront, along with bottles of extra-virgin olive oil flavoured with herbs and olive oil soap. Everything is kept swept, scrubbed and free of litter, and even the water in the harbour is pristine, thanks to the islanders' dedication to avoiding pollution.

With the advent of the tourist industry on Symi, the traditional life is beginning to change. Crops once home-grown on the terraces above the village are being replaced by fruits and vegetables imported from nearby islands, and other produce also comes in from outside. Water, which is in short supply, is bought from Rhodes, and where it was once used for irrigating crops it is now being used for washing machines and bathroom showers. Fortunately, however, the island is saved from excess tourism by preservation rules and a lack of space and water, so that most outsiders can only visit for the day, although once they have sampled Symi's special atmosphere they invariably return.

The classic Mediterranean diet

The most important ingredient in the long and healthy lives of the Symiots is their diet. Symi has its own unique style of cooking, although it has much in common with the classic heart-friendly Cretan diet. The Symi diet is delicious, fulfilling and wonderfully undiet-like.

Not for the Symiots the sad and lonely lettuce of the typical dieter – they enjoy olive oil, fish, succulent tomato sauces, goat's milk cheese, Greek yoghurt and a little meat with their vegetables and salads, all washed down with moderate quantities of wine. The basics, however, still conform to the ideal diet for longevity as outlined in this book, with raw or lightly cooked fruits and vegetables forming the bulk of meals, plenty of the right types of fat, low amounts of saturated fats, and an absence of refined or processed foods.

Olive oil

Extra-virgin olive oil is consumed with everything: bread is dipped into it, vegetables are cooked in it, salads are drizzled with it; even coffee is drunk with it. Olive oil is your heart's friend. It carries vitamins E and A around the body, preventing cholesterol from oxidising and damaging the arteries, and it raises levels of 'good' HDL cholesterol which scours excess fats out of the bloodstream (see Chapter 10 for more on cholesterol).

Extra-virgin olive oil is a 'good' fat that you can eat without guilt; when cardiologist Serge Renaud put 300 heart-attack patients on a low-fat diet and 300 on an olive-oil-rich Cretan diet similar to the Symi diet, the latter group had a 75 per cent lower incidence of heart attack and death within two years than the low-fat group (see Chapter 11 for more on good and bad fats). Olive oil is safe for cooking, as it is more stable than polyunsaturated oils, and is even better used raw in salad dressings.

Olive oil aids digestion by prompting the gall bladder to release bile, clearing undigested food particles and lubricating the gut. It is also anti-fungal, and therefore helps to eliminate candida and keep the gut flora balanced. It protects the gut lining from harm – Symiots drink a spoonful of it neat if they are planning to go out for a boozy evening.

Olive oil can even keep your love life youthful, as it keeps the circulation going to those all-important areas of the body. It is considered by the Greeks to be an aphrodisiac, and newlyweds traditionally ate bread soaked in the first olive oil of the year. As they say in Greece, 'Eat butter and sleep tight, eat olive oil and come alive at night'.

Fruits and vegetables

As for all long-lived populations, vegetables form the main part of the meal in Symi. They are made into mouthwatering dishes with the use of olive oil, lemon, herbs and garlic. Classic Mediterranean vegetables such as artichokes, green beans, stuffed vine leaves, potatoes and Greek salads are all popular staples. Artichokes, delicious with olive oil and lemon, are an excellent tonic for digestion and liver function, and have been found to lower cholesterol levels.

Symiots also love their fruits, many of which are still home-grown, with fig and pomegranate trees decorating the streets and squares, and vines full of sweet bunches of grapes shading the courtyards and doorways. In addition, oranges, apples, lemons, pears and peaches are all imported from neighbouring islands and eaten regularly. Most Symiots eat around double the five portions of fruits and vegetables recommended to us by anti-cancer institutions, so they get plenty of health-promoting fibre and, crucially, antioxidants (see Chapter 7).

Tomatoes

Some researchers believe it could be the humble tomato that is at the centre of the renowned good health of Mediterranean people such as the Greeks and Italians. Tomatoes are the best food source of lycopene, a powerful antioxidant that gives tomatoes their red colour and is the subject of much interest among longevity scientists. In a study published by the *Journal of the National Cancer Institute*, it was found that men regularly consuming high levels of tomatoes reduced their risk of prostate cancer by over a third. Lycopene is also thought to protect against heart disease, as it prevents cholesterol from oxidising and damaging arteries.

Lycopene is fat soluble, and therefore best absorbed when gently cooked in olive oil, as is done with pasta sauces and stews in Symi and other parts of the Mediterranean. Symiots also enjoy tomatoes raw in salads with an olive oil and garlic dressing.

Garlic

Symiots eat garlic with everything – tsatsiki, fish, Greek salad, meat and vegetables are all infused with its potent, uplifting flavour. Garlic, once known as 'the stinking rose', is an incredible superfood that deserves all the praise it gets.

Garlic contains at least twelve different antioxidants, including top players selenium and zinc. It lowers blood pressure and improves circulation, and is antibiotic, antiviral and even good for mental health.[2] Garlic goes bombing through the digestive tract, leaving the corpses of pathogens (*see page 202*) scattered in its wake, and has been found to cut the risk of colorectal and stomach cancer by up to a half.[3] When you use garlic in cooking, heat it gently so as not to destroy the antioxidants, and make sure you also use it raw in salad dressings.

Capers

Symiots have their own unique version of the Greek salad, which they consider to be both better tasting and more nutritious than other versions, partly as it contains capers (*see page 50* for recipe). The sharp, piquant taste of capers is excellent in salads and rabbit and fish dishes; Symiots also sometimes eat capers on their own, including the little stalk and leaves.

Capers are used as a folk remedy for stomach ailments in Greece and are thought to promote longevity. Agapios Monachos, a Cretan writing in the fifteenth century, wrote of the caper that 'it cures the spleen, destroys vermin, heals the haemorrhoids, increases the vitality of the sperm, cures liver ailments and cramps, mobilises the urinary bladder, facilitates menstruation, and prevents rheumatism', and recommended eating one before each meal.

Herbs

All over Symi, the breeze carries a cocktail of herbal smells to greet the nostrils and remind one of dinner. Thyme bushes, with their mauve and lilac flowers, dot the hillsides, while basil, sage, peppermint and spearmint all grow in pots on people's doorsteps.

Herbs are used in most Symiot dishes. Marjoram goes into Greek salads and marinades, rosemary is steeped in wine and olive oil, and mint is used to flavour cheese and lamb dishes.

Herbs are valued as digestive aids and for their antiseptic properties. Sage tea, which is drunk in preference to coffee, is thought to help cure colds and bronchitis and settle the stomach, while lemon balm is used make a home remedy for angina, hysteria and other nervous disorders.

Fish

The best fats of all – the essential fats – come from fish, especially oily fish such as sardines, mackerel, herring and salmon. Like the Okinawans, the seafaring Symiots have plenty of fresh fish to eat, so ensuring an optimum intake of omega 3 fats and their derivatives, EPA and DHA (see Chapter 11).

Most Symiots eat fish at least two or three times a week, the amount recommended by nutritionists. Sardines are one of the more common types of oily fish eaten – they are large and fresh, resembling mackerel rather than tinned sardines. Fish is gently sauteed in olive oil, roasted in the oven or made into succulent soups. Traditionally, Symiots also preserve their fish in salt and eat the salty flesh – not a particularly healthy practice, but since their diet is generally low in salt they seem to get away with it.

Home-made wholemeal bread

Fresh, home-made bread from wholewheat flour is always found on the table at mealtimes in Symi. The bread is dipped in olive oil and accompanies feta cheese, soups, stews, fish and salads, or it is eaten on its own for breakfast. Bread made with wholemeal wheat and sesame seeds is a Symi speciality (*see page 48* for recipe). Wholemeal bread contains fibre, B vitamins, iron, magnesium, zinc and vitamin E (see Chapter 12 for more on whole grains).

Beans

Symiots make stews with beans, tomatoes, garlic, herbs and a little lamb when this is available. Beans are a good source of vegetable protein, and when eaten with a piece of wholemeal bread on the side they provide a complete protein meal with all eight essential amino acids (see Chapter 9 for full explanation). Beans are full of valuable vitamins and minerals, including the B vitamins that are so crucial for metabolism. They contain both soluble and insoluble fibre, which scours excess cholesterol and toxins from the body, and makes them filling and at the same time low in calories.

Lean meat used sparingly

Meat is eaten only in small quantities in Symi, as among all long-lived populations. Organ meats, rabbit, goat and lamb are all popular for stews or roasted with garlic and herbs such as rosemary. Meat was traditionally available only from local herds, and there are no supermarkets on Symi with stacks of cheap, battery-farmed meat as there are in our cities. Meat is therefore reserved for special occasions such as a Sunday dinner. The sheep and goats wander freely around the hilltops of Symi, and they are not treated with antibiotics or hormones, so are lean and organic. Wild animals contain fewer saturated fats and higher levels of essential fats than their battery equivalents.

To eat meat like the Symiots eat it, buy organic, free-range meat, trim off any fatty parts and use it as a special treat only. This will justify the expense of buying organic meat and make it something to really look forward to (for more on why you should limit meat consumption, see Chapter 9).

Organic feta cheese and yoghurt

Like meat, dairy produce is available to the Symiots in moderate quantities only, as it should be in any healthy diet (see Chapter 9). Feta cheese is traditionally home-made from ewe's or goat's milk. It is sliced up and eaten with bread or Greek salad (the word 'feta' comes from the Greek for 'slice', and real Greek feta should be firm enough to slice without being rubbery or crumbly). Sheep's and goat's milk cheeses are easier on the digestion than cow's milk products, and the cheese on Symi is also made from organic, unpasteurised milk, so it still contains the enzymes necessary for digestion that are killed during pasteurisation.

Live yoghurt made from local cow's milk (organic of course) is another traditional product. Symi yoghurt is not low in fat, but it is free of sugar, thickeners and additives. Like the best yoghurts sold in our supermarkets, it contains live cultures that protect our guts from pathogens (*see page 202*) and benefit the digestion. On Symi, yoghurt is eaten either on its own or blended with cucumber and plenty of raw garlic to make tsatsiki.

Wine

Meals in Symi are usually taken with a little red or white wine, or variations on ordinary wine such as ouzo, raki and retsina. Retsina, flavoured with pine resin, is enjoyed by locals as it is a good accompaniment to the strongly flavoured ingredients that are used in Greek peasant cooking such as capers, herbs and salty feta cheese.

Wine drinking is partly credited by cardiologists for the low rates of heart attack in Mediterranean areas. Substances in grape skins (especially red grape skins), such as the anti-oxidants resveratrol and quercetin, protect the arteries from plaque. Wine also contains compounds that dilate the blood vessels and keep the arteries to organs, including the heart and brain, elastic and youthful; moderate wine and sake drinkers have been found to have higher IQs than non-drinkers. Wine may also protect against cancer – when cardiologist Serge Renaud studied 34,000 middle-aged men in France, he found that the death rate from all causes, including heart disease and cancer, was reduced by up to 30 per cent in moderate wine drinkers.[4]

Too much wine, however, increases the risk of cancer, and just one glass daily can increase the risk of breast cancer (see Chapter 1). A generally healthy diet will affect the odds – the long-lived women mentioned in this book drink moderately and have very low rates of breast cancer. Alcohol is a toxin, and some people can tolerate more of it than others. Do not drink it on its own, as it can damage the stomach lining; in Symi, wine is drunk either with meals, or with small dishes of *mezzedhes* such as cucumber and feta, or grilled octopus.

Regular exercise

Symiots are kept fit by having to go up and down the 387 wide stone steps leading up through the village several times a day to do their errands (although someone has had the foresight to build a bar at the level of the 375th step, where people can rest and chat). Traditionally, fishermen had the additional benefits of using oars rather than outboard motors, while herders and farmers were obliged to roam the hillsides in the course of following their herds and tending their crops. Having regular exercise is an important part of the Symi formula for long life and good health (see Chapter 19 for benefits of exercise).

Low stress and happy families

Symiots love living, loving and eating, but they do not gorge themselves on anything. They bask in the sense of well-being that comes from living in a beautiful environment with fresh air and clean soil. Most of them are happy, relaxed and serene, and keep themselves busy and fulfilled, although many of the older people have had to work very hard during their lives.

Symi is often described by locals as being one big neighbourhood, where everyone knows everyone else and people sleep with their doors open without fear of crime. Families are large and loving, so that members benefit from knowing that they have an unconditional support system. Additionally, Mediterranean men such as the Greeks and Italians are able to express their feelings, argue, cry and be more tactile with each other than men in many other cultures; being able to do this lowers stress and is thought to benefit heart health.[5]

Georgios Kokkinos, 96 years old

Georgios Kokkinos still walks down and back up the eighty village steps to do his shopping each month. He describes himself as being in 'a good state of mind' and enjoys an active life, waking at sunrise to do housework and tend the broad beans, onions and garlic in his garden. Georgios believes that the secret of his longevity is that he has worked hard and kept busy. He also believes in God, and feels that close family bonds are a necessary component of long life. 'My favourite time is when my family is all together,' he says.

Georgios loves meat, especially tripe, brain and entrails, but only eats it once a week. He also eats fish two or three times a week, and particularly loves salted fish. He used to eat home-made pasta and home-made bread several times a week. He has yoghurt every night and a little feta or goat's milk cheese every day, and has always eaten a lot of vegetables and salads although he is not so fond of them any more. He drinks about one and a half litres of water daily, and used to drink tea with cloves, sage, cinnamon and rosemary. He has a glass of ouzo every day, and used to have wine on special occasions.

Esmeralda Stavra, 107 years old

Esmeralda Stavra was 107 years old when she died. Her son and daughter-in-law, Manoles and Maria, say, 'Her house was at the top of the village steps, and even when she was 100 years old she went up and down them three or four times a day so that she could sell the feta cheese and yoghurt she made.' Esmeralda was never sick during her lifetime and never went for a check-up with the doctor. Maria says, 'When she died, my mother thought she had just gone to sleep – that's how quietly she went.'

Manoles and Maria believe that Esmeralda's good health was due to hard work and not too much food. 'I think the food has something to do with this,' says Maria. 'There's no sugar, and they don't have diabetes like they do where they eat a lot of rubbish. She had fish about twice a week, but not much meat. She preferred not to eat meat at all, and ate mostly vegetables and salads, with bread, olives, cheese and tomatoes. The vegetables were never sprayed. They don't use butter, only olive oil. She also drank a little bit. She was a very spiritual person – they had fewer worries than we do now.'

SYMI DOS AND DON'TS

Symiots do:

- Eat a diet high in nutrients and moderate in calories.
- Eat plenty of fresh fruits and vegetables from local sources.
- Get plenty of essential fatty acids from fish.
- Use olive oil regularly.
- Eat whole grains rather than refined carbohydrates.
- Eat vegetable protein.
- Drink moderate amounts of wine.
- Get regular exercise.
- Keep busy but mainly stress free.
- Live in a loving, close-knit community.

Symiots don't:

- Overeat.
- Overcook their foods.
- Eat sugar.
- Eat refined or processed foods.
- Eat too many meat or dairy products.
- Smoke.
- Drink much tea or coffee.
- Drink alcohol in excess.

Symi Recipes

RUSTIC BREAD WITH OLIVE OIL AND SESAME SEEDS

Bread is easy and satisfying to make, and it fills the home with a delicious welcoming smell. When you have made it once you will find you will want to make it regularly, and no other bread will taste as good.

Makes 1 large loaf
10 g dried yeast (about 1 tbsp)
2 glasses tepid water
500 g (1 lb 2 oz) whole meal flour (or other whole grain flour)
2 tsp sea salt
Extra-virgin olive oil
1–2 tsp sesame seeds

1. Dissolve the yeast in a glass of tepid water.
2. Mix the flour and salt together and put in a pile on a clean, dry surface. Make a well in the middle and add the dissolved yeast water, a little at a time. Each time you add it, swirl the yeast into the flour using circular movements with four fingers until the yeast is thoroughly mixed in.
3. Keep adding water and mixing together until you have a moist dough. Knead the dough for 5 minutes until it is springy – the Symiots claim that, when done, it should feel like a woman's breast. If the dough is too dry or too sticky you can add more water or flour as required.
4. While kneading, add a little olive oil at intervals (about 2 tbsp in total).
5. Form the dough into a roundish shape and put on a baking tray. Score the top with a knife – this helps it to prove (and

makes it look professional). Cover with a tea towel and leave to prove in a warm place for 40 minutes to 1 hour, until it is roughly double its original size.

6. Punch the air out of the dough and knead for a couple of minutes. Reshape into a loaf and prove a second time for 20–30 minutes.

7. Sprinkle the top with sesame seeds, and bake in a preheated oven at 225° C/435° F/gas mark 7 for about 25 minutes or until done (it should be going brown on the outside, and sound hollow when tapped on the base).

8. Serve warm with a small bowl of extra-virgin olive oil for dipping.

TSATSIKI

This is very quick to make and is a far superior version of the kind of tsatsiki that you can buy ready-made in a supermarket. You can vary the amounts of ingredients according to taste.

Serves 3–4

½ cucumber
2–3 cloves garlic
Small pinch sea salt
350 g (12 oz) Greek yoghurt
1 tbsp white wine vinegar
2–3 tbsp extra-virgin olive oil
1 tbsp chopped mint or dill

1. Peel and grate the cucumber and squeeze out as much of the moisture as possible.

2. Mash the garlic with the salt in a pestle and mortar.

3. Mix together the cucumber, garlic and yoghurt.

4. Slowly stir in the vinegar and olive oil.

5. Add the mint or dill and stir in.

GREEK SALAD, SYMI STYLE

Wait for a summer day, then make this with the freshest, best-quality ingredients you can find and enjoy it out in the sunshine.

Serves 3

2 tbsp extra-virgin olive oil

1 tbsp white wine vinegar

1–2 cloves garlic, chopped small

4 fresh tomatoes, sliced

1 cucumber, sliced

1 onion, sliced thin

15–20 black olives

3 tbsp parsley

1–2 tsp oregano

30 g (1 oz) capers (with leaves and stalk if you can get them)

150 g (5 oz) organic feta cheese

2–3 large fresh sardines (the Symiots salt theirs and marinate them in white wine vinegar first)

Sea salt and freshly ground black pepper

Mix together the oil, vinegar and garlic to make a dressing. Mix together the other ingredients, except the fish, and sprinkle with the dressing. Lay the fish on top and add a little salt and pepper to taste.

SPICY TUNA SALAD

Serves 2–3

1 can (185 g/6 oz) tuna in olive oil
4 free-range eggs, hard-boiled and cut into quarters
50 g (2 oz) capers, chopped very small
100 g (4 oz) gherkins, chopped very small
3 potatoes, boiled and diced
2 onions, sliced very thin
3 tomatoes, chopped
50 g (2 oz) small black olives
5–6 anchovy fillets
1–2 green peppers and 1–2 red peppers, chopped
1 lettuce

For the dressing:

Either (shaken together)
2 tbsp extra-virgin olive oil
1 tbsp white wine vinegar or apple cider vinegar
1 tsp Dijon mustard
1–2 cloves garlic, chopped small
Sea salt and freshly ground black pepper

Or (mixed together)
5 tbsp home-made mayonnaise
1 tbsp mustard
Sea salt and freshly ground black pepper

Make a bed of the lettuce. Mix the ingredients together and put in the middle of the lettuce. Sprinkle with the dressing.

FISH SOUP

This soup has a beautiful rust colour and a succulent flavour –
excellent for a hangover. Have it with a Greek salad and home-
made bread.

Serves 3

For the fish stock:

Fish for boiling, including the heads and bones (turbot, halibut
or monkfish heads and bones are best)

1.2 litres (2 pints) water

1 onion

2 sticks celery

1–2 carrots

2 bay leaves

6 peppercorns

A few stalks of flat-leaved parsley

1 tsp sea salt

For the soup:

500 g (1 lb 2 oz) fish for boiling, filleted (such as fresh sardines or
monkfish – ask your fishmonger for his recommendation)

2 tbsp extra-virgin olive oil

1 onion, chopped

2–3 cloves garlic, chopped

3 sticks fennel, chopped small

2 glasses white wine

2 large tomatoes, chopped small

1 tbsp tomato paste

Juice of 2 lemons

Sea salt and freshly ground pepper

Large pinch saffron

1–2 large potatoes, peeled and sliced into thick slices

A few sprigs parsley

1. To make the fish stock, put all the ingredients in a large pan of water and boil for about an hour until the juice is reduced by half. Strain, throw out the solids, and keep the juice.
2. To make the soup, heat the oil gently in a heavy-based pan and sweat the onion, garlic and fennel. Keep the heat low, add a spoonful of the fish stock, and put the lid on.
3. Add half the fish and stir it around in the vegetables.
4. Add the wine, turn up the heat and cook until the wine has reduced by half.
5. Add the tomatoes, tomato paste and lemon juice, and continue cooking for several minutes.
6. Cover with the fish stock and simmer until the liquid has reduced by half.
7. Taste and add salt, pepper and more lemon juice if desired.
8. Add a large pinch of saffron.
9. Put in the sliced potatoes and the rest of the fish, and cook for about 10 minutes.
10. Garnish with parsley and serve.

BAKED FISH IN WINE

Serves 2–3

1 large fish for baking (use one whole fish such as salmon, trout or
monkfish if small enough)

Sea salt

2–3 tbsp parsley, chopped

1–2 large cloves garlic, chopped

1 lemon

5 or 6 ripe, red tomatoes

2 onions, sliced

1 green pepper, 1 red pepper, 1 yellow pepper, cut into strips

240 ml (8 fl oz) extra-virgin olive oil

1 large glass white wine (for cooking – keep another for drinking)

1. Clean and wash the fish if necessary.
2. Put a little salt on both sides of the fish, stuff the belly with
   the parsley and garlic, then squeeze the lemon over the fish.
   Refrigerate for 1 hour.
3. Put half the tomatoes, onions and peppers in a small baking
   dish in a layer, place the fish on top, then put a second layer
   of the vegetables on top. Pour over the oil.
4. Bake at 200° C/400° F/gas mark 6 for 15 minutes, then baste
   the mixture with the juices. Add the wine, and bake for
   another 15 minutes.

3

Campodimele, village of eternal youth

•

I T IS NOT UNUSUAL to see a ninety-year-old whizzing about on a Vespa among the teenagers or rising at dawn to work in the fields in Campodimele, otherwise known as Europe's 'village of eternal youth'. Campodimele (literally, 'meadow of honey'), a serene hilltop village halfway between Rome and Naples in southern Italy, seems to breed unusually high numbers of death-defying inhabitants.

It is rare for Campodimelani to die before the age of eighty-five, and they often reach their nineties and even sail past a hundred without ever having to visit a doctor. At the last count in 1995, there were forty-eight 90-year-olds, three 99-year-olds and one 104-year-old among the 840-strong population. Yet this is not an old people's resort, but a family-based community where people ranging from one to a hundred years old gather daily in the cobbled piazza to enjoy each other's company. For some unknown reason, men often live longer than women. The oldest male is currently 102 years old – an age that is reached without evoking any particular comment in this haven of health and happiness.

The village, a labyrinth of cobbled streets and stone-walled houses surrounded by a medieval fortified wall, enjoys a panoramic view of the valley below and clean mountain air and fresh sea breezes. Growing beneath are endless olive groves, orchards of fruit and nut trees, and terraces filled with vegetables and grains, as well as grazing areas for cows, goats and sheep. Outside the houses are trellises wreathed in grape vines, and decorative pots of basil, oregano, rosemary and bright orange chilli peppers. Each household has its own plot of land, and work traditionally consists of tending the crops and helping each other bring in the harvests to make olive oil, Parma ham and generous quantities of red and white wine.

For a decade experts have been studying the villagers in an attempt to find the secrets of their longevity. Their findings indicate that this is due to the fresh mountain air, plenty of outdoor exercise, low stress and above all a diet containing large amounts of fresh vegetables. In short, there has not yet been the modernisation, or 'Americanizzazione', as they call it, of lifestyle. In addition, a combination of good diet and healthy living down the generations is thought to have con- tributed to robust genes, giving new-born Campodimelani a useful headstart. The number one killer in the West, heart disease, is not a problem for Campodimelani. According to a study conducted by the World Health Organisation in 1985, even villagers in their eighties have extremely low blood pressure, and a 1995 University of Rome study showed that cholesterol levels in people of all ages are equivalent to those of infants.[1]

Campodimele cooking

Campodimelani eat their food with gusto and relish, and during the day they discuss forthcoming meals with interest and happy anticipation. Ceps and snails in garlic and white wine, artichokes in season with lemon and olive oil, fresh hand-made cannelloni with tomato and wild boar sauce, and salads of freshly picked rocket and lettuce with morsels of delectable home-made goat's milk cheese are all typical fare for the gourmet Campodimelani. Campodimele cuisine has its origins in simple Italian peasant food. Low in salt and high in life-prolonging antioxidants, this type of diet was pounced upon in the 1960s by American nutritionists who declared it to be exceptionally good for health; it is now revered by professional chefs all over the world.

Dishes are based on wholewheat bread and pasta, pulses and large amounts of fresh fruits, olive oil and vegetables grown on fertile, organic soil rich in vitamins and minerals. According to the Campodimelani, the particular essence of their diet is that their food is home grown and home made, and uncontaminated by additives, pesticides or artificial substances of any kind. Soil kept fertile with organic manure ensures that the villagers enjoy top-quality, fresh ingredients that are full of vitamins and minerals as well as flavour.

A perfectly balanced diet

The University of Rome study showed that the Campodimele diet is 'perfectly balanced'.[2] It has a good ratio of protein, fats and carbohydrates, although it has higher amounts of all of these than some of the other diets in this book, with around 100 g of protein, 70 g of fats, and 300 g of carbohydrates eaten daily. Protein tends to come from vegetable sources such as pulses, rather than animals, and requirements for all eight essential amino acids are perfectly satisfied. As a result of low meat intake and high consumption of olive oil and plant foods, the diet is low in harmful saturated fats but high in beneficial monounsaturated fats and essential polyunsaturated fats. Cholesterol intake is not particularly low but, crucially, blood cholesterol levels are low due to a diet that induces high HDL ('good' cholesterol) levels and low LDL ('bad' cholesterol) levels (see Chapter 10). According to study leader Dr Pietro Cugini, Campodimelani also possess a particular enzyme that keeps blood cholesterol levels down.

Campodimelani say that they like to eat and drink 'a little of everything'. The wide variety of produce grown and eaten ensures consumption of the full spectrum of vitamins and minerals, enabling them to work together as they must. The University of Rome researchers found that the vitamins and minerals essential for good health are provided in abundance in the local diet.

Campodimelani eat just enough

There are no supermarkets in Campodimele – any food eaten has to be grown at home – so eating is not done to excess. The University of Rome study showed that women eat an average of 2,200 calories a day and men 2,650 calories, which seems to be an acceptable amount for those who exercise as hard as the Campodimelani do, and they are not overweight (Chapter 6 contains more on the link between low calorie intake and long life). Campodimelani also give their digestive systems an easy time by eating in a relaxed setting – they sit down together for dinner, taking the time to linger over their food and enjoy their delicious cooking.

Fruits and vegetables

Fruits and vegetables are the pride and joy of the Campodimelani, who grow and eat them in great abundance and variety. The wide range of plant foods gives everyone the full quota of fibre and antioxidants required for optimum health. The villagers are wary of fruits and vegetables offered for sale from outside, lest they contain artificial chemicals, and claim proudly that the best food is to be found at home. Because the food produce is collected in season from a very short distance away, the vitamins do not have a chance to disappear by the time they are eaten, and maximum flavour is retained. Vegetables are eaten as salads, or boiled and served alongside other dishes, and are of such good quality that they are delicious just on their own. Some Campodimelani drink the water they have cooked their vegetables in, believing that it purifies the blood.

The Campodimelani enjoy fruits such as apples and pears from their orchards, grapes, and oranges and lemons. Vegetables include delicious Mediterranean varieties such as artichokes, aubergines, cabbage, asparagus, green beans, fennel, cauliflower, rocket, lettuce, peppers, chilli peppers, courgettes, celery, peas and carrots. Verdura, or greens, are considered to be very important for health, and are eaten frequently. Potatoes are also a staple and are used in stews and soups or combined with wheat flour to make gnocchi. Wild mushrooms such as porcini mushrooms are gathered from the mountainside and preserved in vinegar and salt water or used fresh in pasta and gnocchi sauces. Like the Symiots, the Campodimelani eat plenty of tomatoes, which are full of the potent anti-ageing antioxidant lycopene, in pasta sauces, stews and soup dishes.

Garlic and onions

Garlic, both raw and cooked, is used to flavour every kind of dish from salad to snails. A speciality of Campodimele, a small onion called the *scalogna*, which is thought to be especially high in nutrients, is also used frequently. Garlic and onions both help to boost the immune system and protect against cancer, and also protect the heart by keeping the blood from clotting.

Olive oil

Olive oil is poured liberally over salads and used daily in cooking by every household; soups have a dribble of olive oil poured on at the end. The oil, harvested from the olive groves that lie all around the hill, is organic, extra virgin and unrefined, so that it is green and cloudy in the bottle, and full of flavour. Olive oil lowers cholesterol levels, aids digestion and contains antioxidants; it is cited by some people living in the Mediterranean, such as the Campodimelani and the Symiots, as their most precious health commodity.

Whole grains

Fresh wholemeal bread is baked at home from home-grown whole wheat, which is full of fibre, B vitamins and minerals such as magnesium, zinc and iron. Like Symi bread, it is not contaminated with the hydrogenated vegetable oils or extra raising agents used in 'plastic' supermarket breads to make it squashy and quick to rise. You can obtain similar bread from good-quality bakeries and some supermarkets, and it is easy to make at home (*see page 48* for recipe).

Pasta, known as *laina*, is a dietary staple; it is made from durum semolina wheat, salt and water. Pasta is made in sheets from which various shapes are cut, and is cooked fresh with tomato sauce and olive oil or put in vegetable soup with pulses. Pasta is not a perfect food, but it is fairly slow burning and, when made from wholemeal flour, contains B vitamins and minerals. Durum semolina wheat is also easier to digest than ordinary wheat, and may therefore suit some people with wheat intolerance.

Corn is eaten on the cob with olive oil, salt and pepper, or ground into maize (*polenta*). Polenta is readily available in supermarkets and Italian delicatessens in the UK and is very simple to prepare – just add water, cook and cool. It can then be cut into wedges and grilled or lightly fried with olive oil, garlic, basil and tomato sauce.

Beans

Cicerchie beans, which look like a cross between a chick pea and a large kernel of corn, and fagioli beans are used to make substantial soups, added to stews or put in salads with olive oil, herbs and garlic. Cicerchie beans are not available outside Campodimele, but any of the large variety of beans available in our supermarkets and health-food shops can be used as substitutes. Beans are a good source of protein and fibre, and provide some of the essential amino acids we need for growth and immunity (see Chapter 9).

Almonds

Almonds, which grow on trees around the village and are eaten straight from the shell, are another useful source of vegetable protein; they are full of essential fats and vitamin E.

Fish

Anchovies and sardines, an excellent source of youth-promoting omega 3 essential fatty acids, are caught on the coast about twenty kilometres away and eaten once or twice a week, which is the number of times recommended by nutritionists (see Chapter 11 for why you must eat essential fatty acids).

Lean meat used sparingly

Any meat used has to be taken from a household's own stock and is therefore only enjoyed as a treat around once a week, or used in small quantities to flavour stews and soups. The meat is lean, because it comes from roaming animals that are not stuffed with food and hormones to make them fat as they are on battery farms. Chicken is the most readily available type of meat, and chickens fed on seeds also provide free-range eggs containing some omega 3 essential fats (you can buy omega 3 eggs in some UK supermarkets). Other animals eaten by the villagers include goats, lambs, cows, rabbits, snails and wild boar, from which delicious wild boar sausages and pasta sauce are made.

Organic, free-range pig meat is made into sausages or delectable Parma ham. Cured meat is not a healthy source of food, but it is not eaten often by the villagers as it is in short supply. Campodimele hams and salamis are in any case very distant relations of the tasteless, antibiotic-filled fatty variety found in supermarkets in the West. Because meat consumption is low and the meat itself is not fatty, diseases related to the consumption of animal fat, such as heart disease, cancer and countless others, are almost non-existent in Campodimele.

Cheese

Milk taken from sheep, goats and cows is sometimes drunk or made into cheese, which is allowed to mature for maximum flavour and is eaten on its own or grated over pasta. Sheep's milk cheese is the most often eaten; sheep's and goat's milk are easier to digest than cow's milk, of which the Campodimelani only have moderate quantities. Parmesan cheese is not indigenous to Campodimele, and butter is not used – bread is dipped in olive oil instead. The milk is fresh, organic, unpasteurised and free of pesticides, antibiotics and artificial hormones. (As explained in Chapter 9, cheese is not a health food; if you do want to eat it, it is probably best if you confine yourself to a limited intake of organic sheep's and goat's milk cheese.)

Wine

Grape vines grow on trellises outside every house in the village, and each household makes around 300 to 400 litres of white and red wine every year (this is shared around large families, so it does not mean that everyone is drunk on two bottles a day!). Wine, which contains the powerful antioxidants proantho-cyanidins, is taken in moderate quantities, always with food, and sometimes diluted with water. Spirits are drunk only very rarely.

Malt drink

Coffee is drunk by only around a third of the population, and then in small quantities. Some villagers prefer a malt drink, made with barley and milk, in the morning, which is full of B vitamins and considered locally to be better for health.

Water

Recent development has brought water into the village from some distance away, but traditionally the villagers drank pure mountain spring water piped down from nearby Mount Faggeta, source of 'Faggentina' bottled water.

Regular physical exercise

The villagers keep fit by walking up and down the hill, digging crops and chopping wood. Some villagers (including even one or two in their nineties) use bicycles to get up and down the hill, which is very hard work and excellent for heart and lung health. Men, including the octogenarians among them, occasionally hunt wild boar, and everyone enjoys a game of football.

In Campodimele, which is 650 metres above sea level, you can almost taste the clear mountain air, and there is a noticeable absence of cars in the village. Fresh sea breezes from the coast keep the climate temperate, which seems to be a common factor among very long-lived populations. Those of us living in cities do not have such benefits, but even walking in an urban park and taking in some deep breaths will help stir some of the sludge from the lungs.

Low stress

As soon as visitors arrive within the village boundary, they are affected by a sense of deep, penetrating calm. The villagers keep their blood pressure down with a relaxed and positive attitude towards life and an ability to live in the moment. They also take a two-hour siesta each afternoon, and the University of Rome study found that they sleep eight hours a night on average. The study also found that the villagers are remarkably in touch with their natural body clocks, traditionally going to bed soon after dusk and rising at dawn.

Active social lives

There is always some kind of community event going on in Campodimele – five or six generations of the young and old might come out and stand on the walls to cheer on a mountain bike race, or just gather outside their houses to chat and watch life go by. The village even has its own small amphitheatre cut into the side of the hill, which has a performance every night during the summer.

People can be as independent as they like, and older people often live alone, even in their nineties or hundreds. The old and very old do not suffer from the frustrating feeling of dependency on others that is so often experienced in modern society. Despite being independent, no one is lonely, because everyone lives near friends and relatives and socialises with them on a daily basis. There is a sense of reciprocity within the community, with everyone joining in to help each other with the harvest, and if anyone is short of something or old and infirm, their neighbours and family make sure they are provided for.

Giuseppe Sepe, 102 years old

Giuseppe Sepe looks a decade younger than his age. Always smiling and cheerful, he has clear, alert eyes and smooth skin, which he keeps shaven for the purpose of 'kissing the ladies'. Until very recently he would walk up the hill himself to collect his pension; for a month now he has been walking with a stick. According to his daughter Filomena, he eats a lot and enjoys his food.

'I don't know why I've lived so long – you have to ask the God up in the air,' he says. 'Five years ago, I was sick with sore bones, but that's the only time I've been to the doctor.' About his diet, he reveals, 'I eat what there is – corn one day, pasta the next, beans the next. I've never smoked, and I used to drink wine. I couldn't eat the modern food we have here today. We've always grown and eaten our own vegetables. There would be one big plate in the middle of the table at meal times, and everyone got just enough – when it was finished, it was finished.'

Quirino De Parolis, 94 years old

Quirino De Parolis stands at his front door, joking and chatting with visitors. 'I don't feel too bad today,' he laughs. 'I live each day as it comes – I am a joyful man.' Quirino lives by himself and is quite self-sufficient, although he usually eats with relatives. 'When I eat I have a glass of wine and sometimes I'll have a glass of beer,' he says. 'I eat everything – I like meat and have it twice a week, and fish when someone can get it for me. I like figs. I get up each day and have coffee and two biscuits, then I'll walk to the bar and have a talk with my friends. I used to ride my bicycle until I was ninety-two but had to stop when I fell, but it wasn't my fault – there were stones in the road.'

CAMPODIMELE DOS AND DON'TS

Campodimelani do:

- Eat a well-balanced, varied diet.
- Eat plenty of fresh vegetables and fruits, grown organically and locally on nutrient-rich soil.
- Get their essential fatty acids, mainly from fish and nuts.
- Use olive oil regularly.
- Eat whole grains rather than refined carbohydrates.
- Eat vegetable protein.
- Drink moderate amounts of wine.
- Get regular exercise.
- Enjoy a stress-free environment.
- Live in supportive families and have active social lives.

Campodimelani don't:

- Overeat.
- Overcook their food.
- Eat sugar.
- Consume much salt.
- Eat refined or processed foods.
- Eat much meat or dairy products.
- Smoke.
- Drink much tea or coffee.
- Drink alcohol in excess.

Campodimele Recipes

PASTA AND BEAN SOUP

This rich-tasting, full-bodied soup, eaten with a salad, is a meal in itself.

Serves 2

1–2 cloves garlic

3 tomatoes

2 tbsp extra-virgin olive oil

1.2 litres (2 pints) pork or vegetable stock

250 g (9 oz) beans (fagioli or cannellini beans are best), pre-soaked

Chilli pepper (optional)

100 g (4 oz) pork, in small pieces

100 g (4 oz) fettuccine, broken into short strips

2 tbsp Parmesan or other cheese

Basil leaves (to garnish)

1. Sweat the chopped garlic and tomatoes in the olive oil.
2. Add the stock, then the beans, and a pinch of chilli pepper if desired. Put in the raw meat and simmer until the beans are cooked (45 minutes–1 hour), adding more liquid if necessary.
3. Add the fettuccine and cook until it is done (al dente).
4. Serve with a drizzle of olive oil and some grated Parmesan or other cheese. Garnish with basil leaves.

GNOCCHI WITH PORCINI MUSHROOMS

Eat this with a mixed green salad.

Serves 1
150 g (5 oz) gnocchi (preferably freshly made from an Italian
delicatessen, but also available in supermarkets)
1–2 tbsp extra-virgin olive oil
35 g (1½ oz) dried porcini mushrooms, soaked in a little warm water
Large pinch of thyme
1–2 cloves garlic, chopped small
Sea salt
2 tsp parsley, chopped
Chilli pepper
2 tbsp Parmesan or goat's milk cheese

1. Put on a pan of water to boil for the gnocchi. Meanwhile, heat
   the olive oil and add the porcini mushrooms with a pinch of
   thyme. Cook for a minute, then add the garlic and a small
   pinch of salt. Cook for another 2–3 minutes, then add the
   parsley and a very small pinch of chilli pepper.
2. When the pan of water is boiling, add the gnocchi and cook
   for a couple of minutes until they float.
3. Serve with the mushroom sauce, a little cheese and an extra
   dribble of olive oil.

PASTA WITH ROASTED RED PEPPERS

Eat this with a mixed green salad. You can eat the peppers on
toast or on their own instead of with pasta, as here.

Serves 2
4 red peppers
2 tbsp extra-virgin olive oil
1 clove garlic, chopped
Sea salt
200 g (7 oz) penne pasta

1. Grill the peppers until black all over, seal in a plastic bag, leave to cool, then skin and remove the insides. Alternatively – a healthier option – you can roast the peppers in olive oil in a slow oven for 30–45 minutes.
2. Cook the pasta in plenty of boiling water according to the packet directions.
3. Tear the peppers into slices and mix with a generous amount of olive oil, the garlic and a small pinch of salt.
4. Serve immediately with the pasta.

MIXED SALAD WITH SESAME SEEDS AND A GARLIC AND OLIVE OIL DRESSING

Serves 2

For the dressing:
1 tsp mustard
1 tsp vinegar (balsamic, white wine or apple cider vinegar)
1 clove garlic, chopped
2 tbsp extra-virgin olive oil

For the salad:
100 g (4 oz) green beans
100 g (4 oz) broccoli
1 lettuce (lamb's lettuce, lollo rosso, cos – anything but iceberg)
10 black olives
100 g (4 oz) feta cheese, crumbled
Sesame seeds (not a Campodimele staple, but these dramatically enhance the taste of any salad)

1. Make the dressing by shaking the mustard with the vinegar to dissolve it, then add the garlic and olive oil.

2. Steam the green beans and broccoli for about 2 minutes, so that they are still crunchy.
3. Mix together the vegetables and lettuce, then add the black olives and the feta cheese.
4. Gently roast the sesame seeds for a few minutes.
5. Pour the salad dressing over the salad, then immediately add the sesame seeds – they should crackle slightly and give off a delicious smell as they fuse with the salad dressing. Toss and serve.

FETTUCCINE WITH ASPARAGUS

Serves 2

1 bunch (about 150 g/5 oz) asparagus (Campodimelani use thin, wild asparagus; use baby asparagus instead, or else cut the stems into shorter pieces)

200 g (8 oz) fettuccine

2 tbsp extra-virgin olive oil

1 clove garlic, chopped small

2–3 tbsp Parmesan cheese

Sea salt and freshly ground black pepper

1. Steam the asparagus for a few minutes until tender but still reasonably firm. Meanwhile, cook the pasta until al dente.
2. Heat the olive oil with the garlic and toss together with the asparagus.
3. Serve with the fettuccine, with some Parmesan grated over the top. Add a very small amount of salt and a good grind of pepper.

4

Hunza, 'happy land of just enough'

•

H UNZA IS A SUBLIMELY BEAUTIFUL VALLEY high up on the old Silk Route in the mountains of north-east Pakistan, where the great Karakorums meet the Hindu Kush and the Himalayas. Home to about 20,000 people, the Hunza valley forms an unexpected lush green cleft among stark glacial peaks and precipitous rocky cliffs. A glance up and down takes in what appears to be the entire height and depth of the planet's surface: the 7,790-metre, snow-covered Mount Rakaposhi towering overhead, bare walls of rock sweeping downwards, green terraced fields on the slopes beneath and the glacial-blue Hunza River carving its way through the valley floor.

The Hunzakuts who live in the valley are famous for their extraordinary longevity and freedom from illness. They are widely believed to have been the inspiration for the original 'Shangri-La', a fictional land described in James Hilton's novel *Lost Horizon*, whose inhabitants enjoy an idyllic life and ever-lasting youth. During the 1960s and 1970s, a sudden flurry of media interest in Hunza led to exaggerated reports of Hunzakuts attaining such great ages as 140, 150 or even 160 years.

When it was discovered that birth dates were measured against calendar events, such as the invasion of the British in 1892 or the birthday of the Hunza ruler, the Mir, rather than being determined by birth certificates, the 'myth' was 'debunked' and interest in Hunza faded away. Unfortunately, the baby was thrown out with the bath water, because the 'myths' are firmly rooted in fact. Hunzakuts may not live to 140, but a respectable body of research shows that they certainly enjoy levels of health and longevity comparable to the other people featured in this book, and that their diets and lifestyles accord with the same principles.

Before the Karakorum Highway was completed in the 1980s, the occasional visitors to this almost impenetrable land were invariably struck by the long life, good looks and virility of the Hunzakuts. When the eminent physician Sir Robert McCarrison was posted to Hunza in the 1920s, he asked, after a seven-year study, 'How is it that man can be such a magnificent physical creature as the Hunza . . . ?' He wrote, 'these people are long lived, vigorous in youth and age, capable of great endurance and enjoy a remarkable freedom from disease in general'.[1]

Hunzakuts of all ages apparently thought nothing of walking rapidly to the nearest town around a hundred kilometres away, scarcely pausing for breath, while men of eighty were observed playing brutal, vigorous games of polo alongside 'young' men of forty or fifty, and ninety-year-olds were even reported to be fathering children. Visitors particularly noted the cheerful dispositions of the Hunzakuts. In 1960, Dr Jay F. Hoffman wrote, 'Here is a land where people do not have our common diseases . . . Moreover, there are no hospitals, no insane asylums, no drug stores . . . no police, no jails, no crimes, no murders, and no beggars'.[2]

The few doctors to work in Hunza have generally been Western researchers trying to uncover the secrets of the Hunzakuts' good health. Physicians visiting in the twentieth century found that cancer rates were zero, serious illnesses were virtually unknown, and digestive disorders such as ulcers, appendicitis and colitis did not exist.[3]

When cardiologists Dr Paul Dudley White and Dr Edward G. Toomey visited in 1964, they reported in the *American Heart Journal* that among their sample of twenty-five Hunzakut men, who were 'on fairly good evidence, between 90 and 110 years old', not one showed a single sign of coronary heart disease, high blood pressure or high cholesterol.[4]

Doctors working in Hunza today agree that the main causes of premature death have traditionally been accidents involving landslides or falls from the treacherous rock faces. There has been some infant mortality and death from infectious diseases such as tuberculosis and smallpox, but otherwise the average person lives into their eighties in good health, and many people live until their nineties and past one hundred.

Experiments involving the Hunza diet

Doctors have been studying the Hunza diet for decades, but the most famous research was done in 1927 by Dr Robert McCarrison, who carried out some experiments on 1,189 rats in order to discover the Hunzakuts' secrets of long life. He gave the rats a typical Hunza diet consisting of everything apart from the fruits – wholemeal chapattis with a little butter, sprouted pulses, fresh raw carrots, fresh raw cabbage, unpasteurised whole milk, a little meat once a week, and plenty of water for washing and drinking. The rats also had plenty of air and sunlight, and some opportunity for exercise, although far less than the equivalent for the Hunzakuts.

When the rats reached the age of twenty-seven months (the equivalent of fifty-five years in humans), they were examined. Even McCarrison himself was amazed by the results: the rats had no diseases that he could detect, and no infant mortality other than the occasional accidental death. McCarrison also noted that the rats were cheerful of temperament, alert and lived harmoniously together.

McCarrison then compared his Hunza rats with rats fed on other national diets. First he fed a group of 'Bengali' rats a diet consisting of white rice, pulses, vegetables and spices. The rats soon developed diseases of the lungs, nose, ears, eyes, gastro-intestinal tract, urinary system, reproductive system, skin, blood, lymphatic system, nervous system and heart – in short, of every organ in the rat anatomy. They also suffered from hair loss, weakness, ulcers, boils and bad teeth, and in addition became vicious and irritable.

McCarrison fed an even more unfortunate group of rats a typical lower-class English diet of white bread, margarine, sugared tea, boiled vegetables, tinned meats and cheap jams. According to McCarrison, these rats duly contracted 'diseases of the lungs, diseases of the stomach and intestines, and diseases of the nerves – diseases from which one in every three sick persons among the insured classes in England and Wales suffers.' Additionally, he wrote, 'They were nervous and apt to bite their attendants; they lived unhappily together, and by the sixteenth day of the experiment they began to kill and eat the weaker ones amongst them.'

A traditional way of life

The health-giving diet and lifestyle of the Hunzakuts is due to a traditional way of life that, until the building of the

Karakorum Highway in the 1980s, was untouched by the modern world. Traditionally, Hunzakuts have eaten only what they can grow themselves of natural food, unadulterated by additives, sugar or processing methods. There has been no pollution from traffic or heavy industry, and artificial Western products have been absent – the Hunzakuts use glacier water for washing themselves and apricot kernel oil to moisturise their skins, and so avoid soaking their bodies with the harmful chemicals, such as sodium laureth sulfate, which are used in modern personal care products.

With the building of the new road, however, convenience foods such as white flour, refined sugar and cheap cooking oils are starting to penetrate Hunza, along with the increased levels of stress that come with a changing way of life. Now, men of sixty-five remark on their grey hairs and wonder that they are getting them so much younger than their fathers did, and some heart disease and hypertension cases are starting to appear. Cancer has also come to Hunza – local doctors have estimated that rates are at one in a thousand. This is low by our standards, but doctors agree that rates are rising and cannot be wholly explained by better diagnostic techniques.

'The happy land of just enough'

The Hunzakuts do not make themselves ill with overeating, but they get just the right amount of nutrients to keep their systems running perfectly. In her book *Hunza Health Secrets*, author Renee Taylor quotes the Hunza ruler, the Mir, who summed it up by describing Hunza as the 'happy land of just enough'.[5] In other words, they eat a high-nutrient, low-calorie diet (see Chapter 6). When Dr Alexander Leaf studied the Hunzakuts, he found that they ate around 1,900 calories daily, including 50 g protein, 36 g fat (mainly essential fats of vegetable origin), and 354 g carbohydrates.[6]

As a rule, nothing is eaten by the Hunzakuts between rising and doing an initial two or three hours' work in the fields, which gives the digestive system a good chance to wake up before being put to work. Eating breakfast immediately on rising, as most of us do, is not a healthy way to start the day – it is much better to wait for half an hour first, while sipping a drink of hot water and lemon juice to cleanse the system.

Just after the winter, before the new crops are in, the Hunzakuts traditionally had a lean period during which there was very little food for a few weeks. As a result, they had to skip meals, which gave their bodies a chance to break down and expel any undesirable matter, such as diseased cells or cholesterol. Fasting practitioners who have studied the Hunzakuts believe that this annual 'spring clean' is an important component of their excellent health (see Chapter 14 for more on the amazing benefits of fasting). Hunzakuts have the additional advantage that they do not load their bodies with extra toxins from an unhealthy diet or chemicals, as we do.

Life-enhancing compost

Historically, the Hunzakuts are an isolated pocket of healthy people, surrounded on all sides by undernourished, diseased and crime-ridden populations. In farming, they distinguish themselves from their less healthy neighbours by avoiding pesticides and religiously fertilising their otherwise barren soil with carefully nurtured organic compost. As J.I. Rodale wrote in his book *The Healthy Hunzas*, 'The magnificent health of the Hunza is due to one factor, the way in which his food is raised. Of that there can be no doubt'.[7]

Every scrap of organic plant and animal waste is collected and lovingly nurtured into a luscious compost heaving with life-giving vitamins and minerals. The Hunzakuts even put their own faeces back into the land, using it to make an extra-rich organic manure. The result is that the land is continually replenished with what it has lost and produces healthy plants full of essential micronutrients, which are not only good for health, but also full of flavour.

'The land where the apricot is king'

Hunza would not be Hunza without its apricots, which is why it is sometimes called 'The land where the apricot is king'. Apricot trees grow everywhere, filling the valley with pink blossom in the summer. Every family owns several apricot trees, and when a girl gets married, she is often given a tree as a gift by her parents.

In the summer, during apricot season, apricots are eaten as they are, cooked in soup, or puréed with glacier water to make apricot smoothies. Apricots often form a meal of their own – a typical Hunzakut might eat fifty or a hundred in one day, and apricot-eating competitions are frequently held. Apricots are also made into jam, which is spread on wholemeal bread and eaten for breakfast. During the harvest, thousands of apricots are spread out over the flat roofs to dry, adding bright orange patches to the pink and green landscape. The dried apricots are stored over the winter so that people can carry on eating apricots with everything – even puréed with snow to make ice cream.

Fresh apricots are a rich source of copper, iron, potassium, fibre and beta-carotene; when they are dried, the nutrient level is even greater. However, it may be in the apricot kernel, rather than the fruit itself, that the real secret of Hunzakut longevity lies. Apricot kernels are the best-known source of vitamin B17, otherwise known as Laetrile, which has been found to be an effective anti-cancer agent.

Ernst Krebs, Jr., one of the greatest scientists of the last century, said, 'the Hunzas represent a population that has been cancer-free for over 900 years of its existence. This population has a natural diet which supplies on the average between 50 to 75 milligrams of vitamin B17 a day.'[8] Resembling and tasting like small almonds, the kernels are eaten by the handful or ground up with other nuts to make a delicious nut spread or a paste for curries. Hunzakuts also crack open the kernels to extract the oil from inside, which is full of essential fatty acids. The oil has a delectable, marzipan-like taste and is used to make salad dressings, spread over cooked chapattis or drunk on its own. The women also put it on their hair and skins to keep them shiny and soft.

Other sources of vitamin B17, many of which are also eaten by the Hunzakuts, are bitter almonds, macadamia nuts, maize, millet, lima beans, kidney beans, sweet potatoes, linseed, buckwheat, sprouted beans and the chewed seeds of all fruits other than citrus fruits, including apple, pear and grape seeds. Nutritionists advise eating the whole fruit along with the seed, as eating a large amount of the seeds on their own may provide levels of B17 that are too concentrated (although the Hunzakuts do not seem to suffer any ill effects from eating large amounts of apricot kernels).

Cherries, mulberries and walnuts

A high fruit intake, especially during the summer, is a major characteristic of the Hunza diet; there is so much of it around that even the animals eat it. When the Hunzakut wants a snack, he doesn't have a packet of crisps – so he climbs a tree and finds a fruit. Apart from apricot trees, every family has mulberry trees, and most families also have cherry, apple, peach and pear trees. Grape vines grow everywhere, and grapes are eaten fresh or made into antioxidant-rich wine. Whichever fruit is in season at the time is eaten in large quantities, fresh, ripe and raw, so enabling the maximum intake of vitamins and minerals, and the enzymes needed for their proper absorption.

Walnuts are also a dietary staple, a significant factor in the Hunza diet since these are one of the best plant sources of omega 3 essential fatty acids. Walnuts are eaten straight from the shell or ground up to make walnut paste to spread on chapatis along with apricot kernel oil. In winter, they are mixed with dried fruits to make a satisfying fruit and nut cake called *sultancoq*.

Vegetables

Along with apricots and other fruits, vegetables form the bulk of the Hunza diet. Spinach is the most commonly used green leafy vegetable, and is usually eaten with potatoes or chapattis. Hunza spinach is rich in fibre, protein, vitamins and minerals such as magnesium, calcium and iron, as well as being full of flavour. It is sometimes eaten raw in salad, and dried for storage when out of season. Potatoes are another diet staple, although they were only introduced in the 1890s and therefore cannot be credited with being a particular cause of Hunzakut longevity.

Other commonly eaten vegetables include the cancer-fighting cruciferous vegetables, cauliflower and cabbages, and lycopene-rich tomatoes. Root vegetables, such as onions, sweet potatoes, yams, turnips, radishes, and red-coloured carrots full of beta-carotene, are used in vegetable curries and stored in cellars over the winter.

Because of the scarcity of fuel, vegetables are either eaten raw or cooked in only small amounts of water for a short time. Popular salad vegetables include lettuce, cucumber, tomatoes, carrots, sprouts, herbs and radishes. These are sometimes dressed with grape vinegar and apricot kernel oil, but are more usually rinsed in a bit of glacier water or wiped on a leaf and eaten as they are. When vegetables are cooked, the juice left over from cooking is drunk, so that any minerals that have leached out into the water are regained. The thrifty Hunzakuts would never dream of peeling their fruits and vegetables, so they also get all the benefits of the antioxidant-rich skins.

Flavourings

Curries are generally flavoured with a little garlic, chilli or coriander, and are not heavily spiced or salted as they are elsewhere in Pakistan, which makes them more friendly to the digestion. Mint is also used to flavour a Hunza favourite – chapattis made with cheese, onion and apricot kernel oil.

Wholewheat chapattis and other grain products

Chapattis are to be found everywhere in Hunza – people can be seen rolling them out, slapping them between their palms, cooking them on hot stone fires or eating them. The wheat, harvested from the lush green wheat fields in the Hunza valley, is ground up by hand into wholewheat flour, and because the germ and husk of the wheat stay in the flour, the chapattis are an excellent source of fibre, minerals and B vitamins. They are cooked for just a couple of minutes on each side, thus preserving most of the nutrients (see Chapter 8 on raw food). The chapattis are thought to be good for reproductive vigour; this may be because wheatgerm contains vitamin E, which keeps the circulation going to those crucial parts of the body.

Other whole grains used are millet, barley and maize, which are often ground into flour for chapattis. When someone is ill, they are often given bread made from buckwheat, which is a rich source of vitamin B17 and is thought by local doctors to prevent cancer. A particularly nutritious, slightly sweet-tasting bread called *diram pitti* is also made from sprouted wheat, which is eaten on special occasions. Sprouted wheat is both more nutritious and more digestible than ordinary wheat; it is available in health-food shops in the West.

Beans and pulses

The Hunzakuts eat around 50 g protein daily, mainly from vegetable sources such as pulses. Lentils are made into dhal, while black and white, pea-like beans similar to fava beans are used to make flour or added to curries. Chick peas are sometimes ground into flour to make chapattis. Pulses are a useful source of B vitamins, protein and fibre, and are filling without being fattening. Because of fuel scarcity in summer, the Hunzakuts commonly sprout their beans to use in salads. Sprouting can double and even triple the content of certain vitamins and minerals, and it also increases the vitamin B17 content.

Small amounts of organic meat and dairy products

The Hunzakuts love meat, but the animals that they keep are skinny, small and few in numbers. Meat is eaten in small amounts, and only rarely. As a result, the Hunza diet contains very little harmful saturated fat and the toxins from meat that are linked with bowel cancer and other diseases. Their meat comes from cows, yaks, sheep and goats; chickens and their eggs are not used because chickens are liable to wander through the crops growing near the houses. The meat is boiled, rather than fried, which keeps down levels of fat and the carcinogens that are formed by browning meat. Meat from free-range animals feeding on nutrient-rich grasses and other plants contains some beneficial essential fatty acids, unlike meat from fattened, battery-farm animals (see Chapter 9 for more on why you should limit the amount of meat you eat).

Dairy products are eaten occasionally in the form of unpasteurised cow's or yak's milk, yoghurt or *burus*, a delicious soft cheese somewhere between cottage cheese and goat's milk cheese. Butter is also made; this is buried in the ground until it has turned rancid. The resulting pungent butter is not to the average Westerner's taste, but the fermenting process does cause it to teem with beneficial bacteria. Ghee is made by separating the fat and boiling it; the ghee is then used for cooking. Hunzakut milk is unpasteurised, and drinking it may therefore bring with it a slight risk of tuberculosis, but the fact that it is unpasteurised also ensures the preservation of essential vitamins and enzymes that make it healthier and easier to digest.

Glacier water

The Hunzakuts, being engineers par excellence, have a very sophisticated, ancient system of irrigation channels. These cut through the near-vertical rock faces to bring icy pale blue water full of beneficial minerals and silt down from the high Ultar glacier to the valley for irrigation and drinking. In the absence of soft or caffeinated drinks, the Hunzakuts drink up to ten or fifteen glasses of water daily, thus keeping their systems cleansed and hydrated.

Geologists who have studied the Hunza water believe that its low surface tension is beneficial to health, since this enables it to carry nutrients to and toxins from cells efficiently. Low surface tension water is recommended for people who are detoxifying or fasting for this reason. The Hunza water is also naturally low in sodium, and before iodised salt was introduced to the area, Hunzakuts occasionally obtained a little salt by collecting salty soil from the mountain rocks and filtering water through it to make the water salty.

'Hunza water' – a potent red wine

'Hunza water' is a potent, sugar-free red wine made from Hunza grapes and drunk now and then with a meal or on special occasions. 'Special occasions' are frequent in Hunza, ensuring that a moderate amount of antioxidant-rich red wine is drunk fairly regularly. As previously mentioned, low to moderate consumption of red wine is common to long-lived populations and has many health benefits. Alcohol of any kind is not recommended for those at high risk of getting breast cancer, however, as it increases the levels of oestrogen.

Herb tea

Whenever the Hunzakuts feel a little under the weather, they drink a sage-like mountain herb called *tumuru*, once misnamed 'tomorrow tea' by the Western media in its quest for the fountain of eternal youth. *Tumuru* is said to relieve headaches and bring colour to the face.

Plenty of aerobic exercise

Apart from leaping nimbly about the mountains throughout the day and clearing large boulders from the roads (where they are often deposited by landslides), the Hunzakuts enjoy various leisure activities that involve vigorous exercise. Their most popular traditional sport is polo, although nowadays this is mainly played in Gilgit, the town just outside the Hunza valley. Theirs is a fast and brutal version of the game: a goat's head was originally used instead of a ball, the horses gallop at extreme speed, there are no rules and blood is likely to be shed. The party-loving Hunzakuts also consider themselves to be superior dancers, and young and old alike love to perform their fast and furious dances at every possible opportunity.

Living for the moment

The Hunzakuts are not innocent natives living in a state of ignorant bliss. They embrace their own liberal form of Islam and, thanks to their ruler, the Mir, have traditionally enjoyed superior levels of education. However, due to their traditional lifestyle they are concerned mainly with matters of the present, such as digging the fields, cooking supper, playing, praying or just contentedly existing in their magical surroundings. Stressful matters such as mortgages, death, bills, taxes or commuting to work by public transport have never been a problem for them. They work enthusiastically and accomplish much, but are tortoises rather than hares, and take breaks when necessary. When asked about their existence, most Hunzakuts describe it as 'a wonderful life'.

Family structure and respect for elders

The Hunzakuts live in extended families that provide a loving, accepting environment. Crying babies and other 'needy' family members are shared out among everyone, so that all in a family give a little and everyone gets plenty. The elderly are respected rather than sidelined, and therefore have a strong sense of purpose in life. They look particularly dignified, with their hair curled up at the back and their big moustaches, and anyone passing them is expected to be first to offer a greeting. In Hunza, the later years are something to look forward to, and are referred to as the 'rich' years.

Jannat Gul, 96–100 years old

Jannat Gul ('flower of paradise') is aged somewhere between ninety-six and a hundred years. She measures her age according to the 1922 visit of the Aga Khan III's brother when, she says, she was in her late teens or older. The most striking thing about Jannat is her infectious spirit. She laughs, jokes and punches her great-niece playfully. 'When I want to go out my son tries to stop me, fearing that I might get hit by a car,' she says. 'I say to him, "Why should you worry when my vision is perfect, and I have no problem with my legs or knees?" I don't even get headaches.'

When asked how she has kept in such good health, Jannat replies, 'I used to drink a lot of apricot oil. I eat bread at most meals, and in summer I eat a lot of fruit – mulberries, apricots, peaches and grapes. We only eat meat in winter. We never used to have tea, only hot apricot juice. My husband was about eighty-six or eighty-seven when he died – he used to eat sprouted wheat and apricot kernel oil.' Jannat stops talking to burst into fits of giggles. 'In my opinion, the secret of my longevity is God's kindness, but I've worked hard and eaten well.'

HUNZA DOS AND DON'TS

Hunzakuts do:

● Eat moderate portions of food that are naturally low in calories.

● Eat fresh, organic, local produce grown on nutrient-rich soil.

● Eat large amounts of raw fruits, especially apricots.

● Obtain essential fatty acids from apricot kernel oil and nuts.

● Eat whole grains rather than refined carbohydrates.

● Drink moderate amounts of wine.

● Drink herb tea.

● Get regular aerobic exercise.

● Enjoy living for the moment and remain mentally active throughout their lives.

● Live in loving extended families.

Hunzakuts don't:

● Overeat.

● Eat sugar.

● Consume much salt.

● Eat refined or processed foods.

● Overcook food, which would result in lost nutrients.

● Eat much meat or dairy produce.

● Smoke.

● Drink tea or coffee.

● Drink alcohol in excess.

Hunza Recipes

Note: traditionally, the Hunzakuts use crushed apricot kernels and their oil for cooking; you can use extra-virgin olive oil instead.

PORRIDGE OATS WITH ALMONDS AND APRICOTS

For a cholesterol-lowering, beta-carotene-raising breakfast, make porridge oats with water and soya milk, stir in a spoonful of honey, and sprinkle almonds and apricots over the top. Try to get the dark orange organic apricots – these contain the most nutrients and are by far the best-tasting apricots you can buy (you can obtain Hunza apricots in health-food shops, but these will have been whitened and are not quite the same as those eaten by the Hunzakuts).

CRUDITÉS

The Hunzakuts don't often bother with salads, but they eat a lot of raw vegetables. They just pick a carrot or cauliflower, wipe off the soil, and eat it as it is.

Instead of eating crisps and salted nuts with your pre-dinner glass of wine, eat cut-up pieces of raw vegetables such as carrots, cauliflower, cucumber and celery, dipped in hummus or guacamole.

CHAPATTIS

Hunzakuts eat these at almost every meal, and they also double up as spoons. They go well with the stew, spinach and dhal recipes below.

Makes 5 chapattis

375 g (15 oz) whole grain flour such as wheat, rye, millet or
buckwheat flour
Water

1. Mix together the flour and water to make dough and knead
   for 5 minutes.
2. Take a small handful of dough and mould into a sphere. Roll
   out with a rolling pin to make a small, circular shape. Slap the
   dough from palm to palm to enlarge and thin it (this may
   take a little practice).
3. Heat a heavy-based frying pan, then cook the chapatti for a
   minute or two on each side. Lubricate the pan with a little
   olive oil if necessary.

SPINACH WITH ONIONS AND FETA

Serves 2

700 g (1 lb 8 oz) spinach, washed and chopped
1 large onion, chopped very small
2 tbsp extra-virgin olive oil
100 g (4 oz) organic feta cheese

1. Steam the spinach for 1–2 minutes, then drain.
2. Gently cook the chopped onion in the oil for a few minutes.
   Add the spinach and cook for 1–2 minutes.
3. Serve with a little cheese crumbled over the top.

DHAL WITH LEMON AND CORIANDER

The Hunzakuts crumble home-made brown bread into their
dhal; alternatively, you can eat it with brown rice. Using either
combination makes this a complete protein meal (see Chapter 9).

Serves 2

200 g (7 oz) lentils (any colour – the Hunzakuts use brown, black or yellow lentils)

1 large onion, shredded

2 tbsp extra-virgin olive oil

3 tomatoes, chopped very small

2 tbsp tomato paste

2–3 fresh green chillis, chopped small

2 tsp garam masala or curry powder

Sea salt (optional)

2 lemons

1 bunch coriander, chopped

1. Wash the lentils well. Place in a pan with 500 ml (16 fl oz) water, bring to the boil and cook for about 15 minutes until soft but not mushy.
2. In the meantime, use a heavy-based pan to gently cook the onion in the olive oil. Add the tomatoes, tomato paste, and chillis and cook for a few minutes. Add the garam masala or curry powder and a little salt to taste.
3. When the lentils are cooked, add them to the mixture and simmer for 5 minutes. Add extra tomato paste and/or water if you want the dhal to be more liquid.
4. Squeeze in the juice of the lemons to taste.
5. Add the coriander at the last minute and stir it in.

LAMB, FETA, AND PASTA STEW

Known locally as *daudo*, this is a favourite dish in Hunza, and is made on special occasions. It does contain meat, but this is boiled and the fat is removed from the meat juices. There is also a healthier, bean-based option (*see below*).

Serves 2–3

200–300 g (8–12 oz) chunks of lamb (about 2 generous handfuls)

1 onion, whole

3 tbsp extra-virgin olive oil

1 onion, chopped very small/shredded

3 cloves garlic, chopped

1 stick celery, chopped very small

6–8 tomatoes, chopped very small

2 tbsp tomato purée

100 g (4 oz) pasta (the Hunzakuts use chapattis cut into small, short strips, like short tagliatelle)

2 tsp oregano or mixed herbs

Sea salt and freshly ground pepper to taste

150 g (5 oz) organic feta cheese (the Hunzakuts use an ancient, crumbly cheese that looks like small rocks and tastes exactly like feta)

1. Boil the lamb in a pan of water with the onion for about an hour, to create stock. Put the meat aside and reserve the stock. Skim fat from the surface of the stock.

2. Gently heat the olive oil in a heavy-based saucepan – you can also add 2 tbsp stock to keep the temperature down. Using a heavy-based casserole dish, gently cook the onion, garlic and celery in the olive oil until soft, but don't let them go brown. Add the meat and cook for a few minutes, then add the tomatoes with the tomato purée and gently cook for 5–10 minutes.

3. Put in enough stock so that the liquid level is about an inch above the solids. Simmer with the lid on for about an hour. Add more juice if necessary (or a glass of red or white wine).

4. Add the pasta and cook until the pasta is al dente.

5. Add the oregano or mixed herbs, and season with salt and pepper to taste.

6. Serve with a little feta cheese crumbled over the top.

BEAN, LAMB AND FETA STEW

This is a variation on the above recipe. Use 350 g (12 oz) beans as well as, or instead of, the lamb (you can use less lamb if you like). Choose brown or red beans, such as kidney beans, and soak them overnight – they go very well with the lamb stock. Add them after step two, and simmer the stew for about 1½–2 hours or until the beans are cooked. You can either include or omit the pasta, whichever you prefer.

Bama, where longevity medicine grows

•

BAMA COUNTY, OTHERWISE KNOWN as Wangang (literally, 'hundreds of mountains'), is an untouched land high up in semi-tropical Guangxi, south-west China. Cut off by the mountains surrounding them on all sides, the people of Bama have no cars, no industrial plants, no supermarkets, and no fast-food joints – just the sparkling clear Panyang River flowing down from the green peaks into the tranquil valley below.

Here, the exceptionally long-lived, vibrant Yao people till the fields and terraces, climbing up and down the mountains to cultivate the crops that provide them with their own special brand of Chinese medicine for long life. Even the horses grazing the nutrient-rich mountain grass are known to live extra-long lives here. The World Health Organisation recently named Bama an official 'hometown of longevity', and a research institute has been established in order to discover the reasons for its people's exceptional good health.

Octogenarians in Bama have the dubious pleasure of looking up to their elders, the nonogenarians, who in turn defer to those aged a hundred and over, of which the area typically has about seventy-four in total, or thirty-four per 100,000 (at times, the number tops even Okinawa's supposed world record). Up to five generations of people often live under one roof, with the oldest joining in the chores and social activities; 100-year-olds have even been known to climb the mountains each day to work the fields, despite the protestations of younger family members. Spirited centenarians can also be found competing against their juniors at the popular folk-singing contests that are held along the banks of the Panyang River every week.

The people of Bama have an exceptionally low incidence of heart disease and cancer, along with low blood cholesterol and robust immune systems. There is no sudden steep increase in the rates of killer diseases after the age of forty, as there is in the West – rather, the people enjoy prolonged youth and vitality to the end. Only 10 per cent of the over-nineties suffer from coronary heart disease, while a mere 4 per cent have been found to have excess blood lipids.[1] In one study, not a single malignant tumour could be found among the population, while in another, the rate was just 4.4 per 10,000 people.[2] The life expectancy in Bama has increased over the last few decades as a result of improved health care, which has reduced infant deaths and deaths from infectious diseases such as tuberculosis.

A natural diet

Bama air is fresh, the water is pure, and the people are kept fit by trekking around the rugged terrain every day. Bama people have happy family lives and a positive outlook on life, and some centenarians have cited 'doing good deeds' and 'close relationships' as the reasons for their longevity. Researchers have also found a slight genetic element, as there tends to be longevity in certain families, with 37 per cent of centenarians having parents over eighty years old.[3] However, genes are thought to be only a minor factor – and genetic inheritance is in any case influenced by the diets and lifestyles of previous generations.[4]

Overall, diet is considered by researchers to be the most important 'secret' of longevity in Bama. Three vegetable-based meals are eaten daily, using home-grown, unrefined organic produce. The diet is low in calories, fat, animal protein and salt, while being high in fibre, complex carbohydrates, vegetable proteins and antioxidants. It also contains the necessary quota of the all-important omega 3 and omega 6 essential fatty acids, derived from the seeds of the hemp plant, as well as omega 3 essential fats from fish caught from the Panyang River.

Bama villagers are cultivators rather than herders, and are therefore unlikely to suffer from colon cancer or any of the other unpleasant ailments caused by a colon clogged with meat. In short, the Bama diet is ideally balanced for optimum health.

When researchers studied the faeces of Bama elders aged between 80 and 109, they found that they contained levels of beneficial *bifidobacterium* that were higher than those of other elderly populations.[5] A gut blooming with friendly flora is a reliable indicator of good general health and diet, and this utopian gut environment is brought about by eating plenty of wholefoods and avoiding popular Western foods, such as meat, sugar and processed foods, which ferment improperly in the colon and feed disease-causing organisms.

Nutrient-rich soil

The soil in Bama is full of all the right kinds of minerals and trace elements we need for optimum health, which find their way through the crops and into the people who eat them. When researchers analysed the soil in Bama, they found that it contained high levels of manganese and zinc, both of which are essential for breaking down food into the nutrients the body needs.[6] Manganese is also valuable to health as it helps make the powerful antioxidant enzyme superoxide dismutase (SOD), which protects our bodies from dangerous superoxide free radicals (see Chapter 7 for antioxidants and free radicals).

The researchers also found that the soil included the right balance of trace elements such as chromium, copper and iron, which are needed in small amounts for such life-lengthening functions as regulating blood sugar, making SOD and building red blood cells respectively. The same study found that villagers who were still fit and well in their nineties had correspondingly good levels of trace elements in hair analysis tests.

Needless to say, the farming in Bama is organic and the crops are devoid of genetically modified (GM) strains or artificial fertilisers and pesticides, which leach the soil of nutrients and cause toxins to accumulate in our cells. The climate is subtropical, so temperatures are always reasonably warm; there is therefore bountiful fresh produce available throughout the year for the locals. Like the other long-lived people discussed in this book, the people of Bama pick their food and eat it soon afterwards, before the vitamins have a chance to deteriorate.

Appetising food

There are certain rules in Chinese cooking: the dishes must be colourful, the aroma must be appealing and the taste must be delicious. When food is lovingly tended and hand-picked so that it is naturally bursting with flavour and beauty, a certain respect is inevitably given to it.

In China, a few extra seconds are always devoted to presenting the food in such a way that just looking at it gets the digestive juices going. This ensures not only enhanced pleasure but also proper absorption and assimilation of the food. It doesn't matter how simple the food is (in Bama, it often consists of little more than cornmeal simmered with vegetables); it can always be presented in an appetising way, for instance by arranging ingredients of different colours around the plate and adding some aromatic herbs.

Vegetables

Sweet potatoes and pumpkins, their orange flesh packed with anti-cancer beta-carotene, are often eaten with corn to provide flavour and texture (as well as colour). Sweet potatoes are lower on the glycaemic index (*see page 173*) than ordinary white potatoes. Another advantage they have over ordinary potatoes is that their flesh is very juicy and does not act like an unquenchable sponge for soaking up butter (organic sweet potatoes are available year-round in our supermarkets and are excellent for baking or mashing).

Tomatoes and peppers, also full of beta-carotene, are frequently used in Bama. Red peppers are one of the richest sources of vitamin C there is, while tomatoes are the only reliable source of the potent anti-ageing antioxidant lycopene (see Chapter 2).

Green leafy vegetables eaten by the Bama people include wild amaranth, an attractive and colourful plant that is similar to spinach. Amaranth contains twice as much calcium as milk, as well as the magnesium needed to get calcium into our bones. It is also high in potassium, phosphorus, folic acid, manganese, iron and the top three antioxidants, vitamins A, C and E. Its seeds, which have a nutty, malty flavour, are available in health-food shops in the West – these can be combined with brown rice or corn to make a complete protein meal, or used to make pasta or bread (see Chapter 12 for more on whole grains).

Vegetables in Bama are not stir-fried or deep-fried with batter and monosodium glutamate, as they are in the average Chinese restaurant in the West. Instead, they are simmered for a short time in hemp-seed broth, which ensures that they retain most of their nutrients and that the meal contains beneficial essential fats, rather than harmful cooking oils (see Chapter 11).

Fruits

The Bama people grow fruits such as bananas, guavas, grapes and pears, all of which are eaten straight off the tree, fresh, ripe and bursting with antioxidants, enzymes, fibre and other nutrients that are essential for a long life. They are fortunate to have such a resource: most of us don't. We should nonetheless eat fruits regularly, and treat ourselves to some local organic produce now and then even if we cannot afford to buy it all the time.

Hemp

One of the main ingredients for long life in Bama is the seeds of the hemp or *Cannabis sativa L.* plant, a cousin of the better known *Cannabis indica* plant. Unlike its relative, the hemp grown in Bama does not have any psychoactive properties – the villagers get those from their sake and snake wine (*see page 102*) instead.

The hemp plant is very adept at soaking up vitamins, such as B vitamins, and minerals such as magnesium and zinc. Crucially, hemp seeds contain a good balance of the essential fatty acids omega 6 and omega 3 (in a ratio of 3:1), which are needed by every cell in our bodies. Hemp is also a complete protein, as it contains all eight essential amino acids. It has been used as a folk remedy in Asia, Russia and Eastern Europe for thousands of years.

Hemp pasta, which is sold in health-food shops in the West, is a delicious alternative to ordinary pasta. It is quick and easy to cook, full of flavour and goes with most pasta sauces. You can also get hemp flour, so you can even make 'cannabis cookies' that are safe for your children to eat! Hemp is gluten-free, so it is ideal for those with gluten intolerance or coeliac disease, and it is easier on the digestion than some grains. Hemp seed oil is also sold as a beauty product and is said to improve the elasticity and lustre of the skin.

The hemp that grows all over the slopes of the Bama mountains is harvested for its seeds, which are dried in the sun, ground into a paste and stirred into pots of clear mountain water. This creates a nutritious milky emulsion that is used as a kind of oily broth in which to cook vegetables, or made into *houmayou*, a soup that is eaten once or twice daily. The seeds are also eaten just as they are, with their essential fats in their purest, most raw state preserved.

Corn

Corn is the staple crop in Bama and can be seen everywhere in the county, growing on the mountainside, hanging up to dry in the sun or being hand-milled into maize. Every day the people of Bama hang up large iron pots by their fires; the maize is stirred into them with big wooden poles and turned into the Bama equivalent of Italian polenta. Extra corn is also fermented and made into corn wine.

Corn is not actually a superfood, but it seems to work for the people of Bama as part of a balanced diet that is generally rich in nutrients. The fact that the corn comes from nutrient-rich soil adds to its health-promoting properties. Recent research from Cornell University has revealed that corn is unusual in that it has higher levels of antioxidants when cooked than when raw.[7] Cooked corn also releases ferulic acid, a phytochemical that is thought to have anti-cancer properties. Additionally, the soluble fibre in corn helps stall the ageing process by regulating blood sugar levels and lowering cholesterol.

Brown rice

Brown rice is grown in the bottom of the valley by the river, and those who live there supplement their corn with rice, which is sometimes made into a porridge called *conjee*. This may explain why a majority of the centenarians (62 per cent of them) is found in this part of Bama.

Brown rice is an excellent source of both soluble and insoluble fibre, as well as nutrients such as magnesium, iron and B vitamins. It wards off colon cancer by getting the stools moving and cleaning out environmental toxins, and protects you from heart disease by lowering cholesterol levels. It is also thought to boost the reproductive system and to promote sexual and mental vigour.

Fresh fish and small amounts of animal protein

Fresh fish is caught in the Panyang River and provides locals with a healthy source of protein containing omega 3 essential fatty acids. The diet also contains some animal protein in the form of eggs and meat, but only in moderate quantities, and all from the lean, organically fed animals that roam the mountainside.

Beans

The Bama diet contains ample amounts of vegetable protein from beans and pulses (see Chapter 9 for why you should eat vegetable protein). Bean varieties eaten include lima beans, mung beans and soya beans.

- Mung beans are excellent for sprouting, which raises their nutrient levels, especially those of calcium, potassium and B vitamins.

- Soya beans, which are fermented into tofu, help balance hormones to ward off cancers such as prostate and breast cancer, both of which are virtually non-existent in Bama.

- Soya is a complete protein (see Chapter 1) – other beans contain some essential amino acids and should be combined with grains such as brown rice for a complete protein meal.

Beans raise levels of 'good' HDL cholesterol (*see page 150*) to improve circulation and protect against heart disease. They are also thought to be cancer-protective, as they contain fibre to clean out the intestines, absorb toxic waste and prevent constipation. They are useful for dieters as they give a feeling of fullness without the calories and take energy to digest, so that they have a 'negative calorie effect'. The fibre in beans also helps to steady blood sugar levels, so keeping down levels of age-promoting insulin and helping to prevent diabetes.

Snake wine and sake

The people of Bama are partial to a drop of snake wine – fermented rice or corn wine that is actually bottled with real snakes preserved in the alcohol. More significantly healthwise, some villagers sip fermented rice wine, or sake, from glazed bowls in moderate quantities throughout the day. Some types of alcohol, including sake and wine, have health benefits when drunk in moderation. Sake can be found in any oriental supermarket in the West – heat it up gently and sip from a tiny earthenware mug in winter to warm you up.

Mountain spring water

Bama villagers get their water for cooking and drinking from the pure, clear, Panyang River that flows into the valley. Panyang water has been found to be high in the manganese and zinc our bodies love and need. If you buy mineral water, check levels of these minerals and try to avoid waters that are high in sodium. Alternatively, you can use steam-distilled water, which efficiently removes unwanted substances from the body.

Herbs

Herbs, which aid digestion and have antiseptic properties, are often used to flavour Bama cooking and are also taken as folk remedies. Two popular herbs used are ginseng and astragalus, both of which can be obtained in health-food shops in the UK. Ginseng is very popular in the Far East as a general tonic for weakness and fatigue, and it also has anti-inflammatory properties, making it useful for treating conditions such as rheumatoid arthritis. Astragalus increases metabolism, combats fatigue and is an excellent tonic for the immune system (see Chapter 15 for information on the immune system).

Life-long physical activity

Thanks to the mountains surrounding them on four sides and the fact that they have no cars, the people of Bama get plenty of aerobic activity. The fact that they live around 1,400 metres up in clean, oxygen-rich mountain air enhances the experience, of course.

Couch potato syndrome is unknown in Bama – children have to climb the mountains to get to school, adults have to climb up and down them all day to tend their crops, and men enjoy hunting and archery even when they are in their eighties. The hard physical work involved in everyday life gives the people strong bones and muscles, including the heart muscle, and is no doubt an important factor behind their excellent health.

Folk singing and other 'mental gymnastics'

Bama people do not have hurried, stressful lives, but they always have something to get up in the morning for. No one, young or old, is ever made to feel redundant. Mahjong, chess and calligraphy are included in the leisure activities, and there are always household chores to be done.

The favourite pastime is folk singing, which has been enjoyed in Bama for the last thousand years. Every week there is a singing fair at Jiazhuan town in the Panyang River Valley. Up to a thousand people gather along the river banks to cheer on the competitors, who range from children to hundred-year-olds. Singing contests are partly a social activity, and are also considered by locals as a means of keeping their brains alert and youthful, since they are required to pit their wits against each other by keeping the crowd entertained with impromptu songs. Researchers studying longevity in Bama believe that the folk singing promotes health and long life by relieving stress, keeping the brain active and boosting the immune system.

Happy families

There are no old people's homes or retirement villages in Bama – young and old mix together, with up to five generations often living under one roof. Researchers have found that the majority of the very long-lived people in Bama live harmoniously in large families of seven or eight people, and in a survey of those aged over ninety it was found that they all lived with their families.[8] One study revealed that one person had recently married at the age of ninety-seven.[9] The same study found that most of the very old – barring those who had recently lost a close relative – were happy and contented.

Huang Buxin, 101 years old

Huang Buxin is typical of many Bama super-centenarians. He says that he is very happy and contented, and considers himself to be in excellent health. Having stayed fit from walking over the mountains all his life, he still does house-work every day and goes on daily outings. Although he lives with his family, he bathes, dresses, goes to the toilet and eats without any help. He has brown rice with almost every meal; it is accompanied by tofu and other beans, as well as by small amounts of fish, meat and eggs. He also has fresh fruits almost every day. He rarely eats sugar or salt, and avoids smoking and drinking.[10]

BAMA DOS AND DON'TS

Bama people do:

- Eat a diet that is high in nutrients and low in calories.
- Eat plenty of fresh vegetables and fruits, grown organically and locally on mineral-rich soil.
- Get essential fatty acids.
- Eat whole grains rather than refined carbohydrates.
- Eat vegetable protein.
- Drink moderate amounts of sake.
- Drink plenty of water.
- Get regular exercise.
- Keep their minds active.
- Have low stress levels.
- Live harmoniously in extended families.

Bama people don't:

- Overeat.
- Overcook their food.
- Eat sugar.
- Consume much salt.
- Eat refined or processed foods.
- Eat animal products.
- Smoke.
- Drink tea or coffee.
- Drink alcohol in excess.

Bama Recipes

SWEET POTATO SALAD

This is an easy recipe, which makes a very good multi-coloured antioxidant lunch (see Chapter 7 for more about antioxidants and coloured foods).

Serves 2
1 baked organic sweet potato
Green salad leaves such as lamb's lettuce, rocket, watercress, cos lettuce or spinach
1 cooked beetroot, sliced
2 tomatoes, thinly sliced
1 avocado, sliced
Handful of basil or coriander leaves, chopped
10 black olives, sliced
Handful sesame seeds
Olive oil and Balsamic vinegar dressing

1. Mix together the ingredients, except for the sesame seeds, and add the salad dressing but do not toss.
2. Heat the sesame seeds in a dry pan for two or three minutes, then add to the other ingredients and toss.

SWEET POTATO AND CARROT SOUP

This is an excellent beta-carotene-rich soup, perfect for winter. The Bama people do not use cardamom or cumin in their cooking, but I have added them because they taste good and have their own health benefits. You can also make this soup with pumpkin.

Serves 2

2 or 3 sweet potatoes
4 or 5 large carrots
2 tbsp extra-virgin olive oil
1 tsp cumin powder
Pinch ground cardamom seeds
850 ml (1½ pints) chicken or vegetable stock

1. Peel and chop the sweet potatoes and carrots.
2. Heat the olive oil in a heavy-based pan and add the sweet potatoes and carrots.
3. Add about a teaspoon of cumin powder and a pinch of ground cardamom seeds, stir in and sweat the mixture gently for a few minutes.
4. Add enough stock to cover the vegetables and simmer until they are soft.
5. Put in a blender and blend – if the soup is too solid, you can add more stock.
6. Return to the pan for a few seconds just to heat the soup through, then serve.

BROWN RICE WITH HEMP SEED

Hemp seed is a versatile food that you can add to almost any dish, such one based on lentils, bread or polenta, or a dip or salad. You can use either hulled or non-hulled hemp seed for this recipe – the non-hulled variety makes the dish quite crunchy. Hemp seed is available from health-food shops. See page *285* for suppliers.

1 onion, chopped small
1 tbsp extra-virgin olive oil
300 g (11 oz) cooked brown rice
75 g (3 oz) hemp seed
2 tbsp soy sauce

1. Sauté the onion in the olive oil for 5 minutes.
2. Add the rice and heat through.
3. Remove from the heat and add the hemp seed and soy sauce.

HEMP PASTA WITH PESTO

Hemp pasta is delicious and very versatile – it goes well with any pasta sauce. Hemp pasta and hemp pesto are both available from health-food shops and some supermarkets.

Serves 1
150–200 g (5–7 oz) hemp pasta
1 tbsp basil or hemp pesto

1. Boil the pasta for the length of time specified on the package (this varies according to the shape of pasta). Drain and return to the pan.
2. Add the pesto, stir and heat through.
3. Serve with a salad.

GRILLED POLENTA WITH SPINACH

There is no Parmesan cheese in Bama, and although it isn't a health food; it does go very well with polenta – use organic cheese if possible.

Serves 1–2

100 g (4 oz) polenta flour
570 ml (1 pint) water
3 tbsp grated Parmesan cheese
Sea salt and freshly ground pepper
2 tbsp extra-virgin olive oil
400 g (14 oz) spinach
1 garlic clove, chopped

1. Bring the water to the boil in a heavy-based pan.
2. Slowly pour in the polenta in a steady stream, whisking it at the same time. Turn down the heat as low as possible and simmer very gently for a few minutes (cooking times vary, so refer to the instructions on the packet).
3. Stir in the Parmesan cheese, a little salt and pepper to taste.
4. Transfer to a small, shallow dish and leave to cool.
5. Cut the polenta into wedges, and brush a little olive oil on either side.
6. Grill the polenta wedges for a few minutes on each side until they start to go golden.
7. Meanwhile, steam the spinach for 1 or 2 minutes, until just wilted.
8. Heat the olive oil in a pan, add the garlic, cook for a few seconds, then toss the spinach in the pan for a few seconds.
9. Serve with the polenta and a few extra shavings of Parmesan cheese.

II

The fifteen secrets of living longer

This section describes the fifteen 'secrets' of living long - and staying young - which the five longevity hot spots in the world have in common. Each chapter explores a specific dietary or lifestyle habit and explains how you can incorporate it into your own life.

chapter

6

Eat exactly what you need

•

THE LONG-LIVED OKINAWANS, SYMIOTS and others described in Part I all have one very important thing in common: they eat a diet that is *rich in nutrients* but *low in calories*. Their food consists of moderate amounts of fresh produce in its natural, unaltered state, such as fruits, vegetables and whole grains. It is therefore rich in vitamins, minerals, protein, fibre and beneficial fats. It is low in saturated fats such as meat and cheese, and low in refined carbohydrates like white flour and rice, which are both devoid of nutrients and high in calories. In short, the populations discussed in this book eat *exactly what they need and no more*.

This way of eating is known by longevity scientists as a 'high nutrient, low calorie' diet, or 'calorie-restricted' diet. As discussed below, dramatic experiments have revealed the amazing effects of such a diet on health and lifespan. The Okinawans are thought to have a near-perfect example of this type of diet: their diet is exceptionally well balanced and provides an average of only around 1,300 to 1,500 calories per day. The populations in the other four regions consume between 1,600 and 2,700 calories daily, which is a very acceptable amount, particularly considering how much exercise they take (the US male average daily intake, by comparison, is 3,300 calories – many of which are just empty calories).

Extending lifespan with a high-nutrient, low-calorie diet

The maximum lifespan of human beings is considered to be about 120 years, with the longest life ever recorded being that of Frenchwoman Jeanne Calment, who died aged 122. Tests on laboratory animals indicate that our maximum lifespan could be extended even further than this, to 130 or even 140 years. The only known way of doing this is by eating a high-nutrient, low-calorie diet.

Eating a strictly calorie-restricted diet might sound like too much of a sacrifice, but you can create your own moderated version and get many of the benefits. Eating this way does not mean picking at bits of celery while fantasising about cheese-burgers (as does going on a diet). It means habitually avoiding excess and the discomfort that comes with it, and giving the body exactly what it needs to run at peak efficiency, like a well-oiled machine. You have been created with an inbuilt potential lifespan, and to a large extent you can choose to either last out the time that has been allotted to you, or hasten the end with overuse. By eating food that has a high amount of nutrients and is relatively low in calories, you can not only live longer but also feel and look younger for longer.

Getting younger by eating less

By eating just enough but not too much, you can slow down or even reverse the ageing process, and it is never too late to start. This process was exemplified in the 1500s by Louis Cornaro, a Venetian nobleman, who wrote down his experiences in his book *Discourses on the Sober Life* (*How to Live to 100 Years*). Cornaro enjoyed a hedonistic lifestyle and overindulged in food and drink until the age of forty, by which time he looked like an old man. He was afflicted with gout, colic and a continual fever, and was told by his doctors that he only had months to live.

Yet Cornaro died at 102, sitting up in a chair and without pain. At ninety-five he wrote, 'O, how glorious is this life of mine, replete with all the felicities which man can enjoy on this side of the grave! . . . How different from the lives of most old men, full of aches and pains and foreboding, whilst mine is a life of real pleasure, and I seem to spend my days in a perpetual round of amusements.'

How did he do it? Firstly, Cornaro simplified his diet so that it included only foods that he found easy to digest, and secondly, he drastically reduced his food intake to a mere twelve ounces of solid food daily, along with fourteen ounces of light wine each day with his meals. He achieved spectacular results, yet his diet was not particularly nutritious (and it is not recommended that you follow it!). What, you may ask, could happen if his methods were to be combined with a diet that is optimally high in nutrients?

A unique experiment

Dr Roy Walford has fed a high-nutrient, low-calorie diet to various animal species in thousands of tests, with extraordinary findings. On this type of diet, three-year-old mice, which would normally be grey, arthritic and shrivelled, look and test as healthy and agile as one-year-old mice, rats live 60 per cent longer lives than usual and fish enjoy (if only they knew it) a life extension of 300 per cent.

Dr Walford's research with humans suggests that you can enjoy the same benefits as his record-breaking rodents. In 1991 Dr Walford tested the low-calorie, nutrient-dense diet on himself and six other men and women in Biosphere 2, a closed ecological space in Arizona. For two years, the Biospherians ate nothing but fruits such as figs, guavas and papayas, organic, whole cereal grains, nineteen types of vegetable, pulses and small amounts of lean meat, eggs, fish and dairy products. For the first five to six months, they ate approximately 1,800 calories each per day; this was gradually increased to 2,200 calories for the rest of the two-year period. The Biospherian diet had rapid and spectacular results.

- The participants' blood pressure dropped from an average of 110/75 to 90/58 after three months, and blood cholesterol levels fell on average from 191 to 123 over six months – a fall more dramatic than any caused by a pharmaceutical drug.

- All the men and women had healthy drops in blood sugar levels unprecedented in drug trials, with fasting blood sugar levels falling from 94 to 65 for the men and from 90 to 68 for the women (an important factor in anti-ageing, see Chapter 12).

- Two of the participants who had severe acne at the start of the study rapidly developed clear skin.

- All of them looked trimmer and more vital.

- They all had greatly increased energy levels.

- Excess weight fell off them and stayed off, with the men losing an average of 33 pounds and the women losing 17 pounds.

Measuring your real age

The various bodily changes experienced by the Biospherians showed that not only did they become *healthier*, but they also actually became *younger* over the course of two years. In effect, they had reversed time by following a high-nutrient, low-calorie diet. In order to understand how this works, think of yourself as having two different ages: your *chronological age*, which is how many birthdays you have had; and your *biological age*, which you could call your 'real' age.

Real age can be measured by various 'biomarkers of ageing'. These are not to be confused with 'biomarkers of health', which overlap but are not identical. Biomarkers of health take into account illnesses such as atherosclerosis or liver cirrhosis, which do not indicate the rate at which you are ageing per se. Biomarkers of ageing, on the other hand, measure the overall rate of ageing of the whole body. Biomarkers of health can be affected by various specific factors such as cutting out fat or taking exercise, but the only known way of influencing biomarkers of ageing is with a high-nutrient, low-calorie diet. In his book *The Anti-Aging Plan*, Roy Walford outlines some useful biomarkers of ageing, such as the amount of air that can be breathed in and out rapidly in one very deep breath, immune system health and blood sugar levels.[1]

How old are you *really*?

If you want to measure your rate of ageing (or unageing), you can ask your doctor to perform tests using biomarkers of health and ageing. Find a sympathetic doctor who knows about nutrition and ask them to measure your 'before' and 'after' cholesterol levels, blood pressure, immune status, vital lung capacity and fasting blood sugar level.

At home, you can try the Static Balance test. Stand on one leg, shut your eyes and see how long it takes before you lose balance. According to Roy Walford, if you are twenty or younger you should be able to stand for any length of time; if you are forty, around twenty-five seconds; if you are fifty, about ten seconds, and not at all if you are eighty. Don't worry, however, if you fall over straight away. The test is not perfect, and other variables, such as fitness and practice, will affect the outcome.

Avoiding cancer and other illnesses

No method has been found to reduce overall cancer risk as much as calorie restriction does. In studies, mice were inbred to be susceptible to certain types of cancer and then fed either a calorie-restricted diet or an ordinary diet. Only 2 per cent of those on a calorie-restricted diet had breast cancer compared with 40 per cent of those on the ordinary diet, and only a fraction of those on the former diet got other types of cancer compared with those in the latter group.[2] Walford and other scientists see no reason why these findings should not apply to humans. A 1995 study published in the *New England Journal of Medicine* found that overweight women died earlier than underweight women, particularly from cancer or heart disease, and that the lowest mortality rates were among women 15 per cent below the average US weight.[3]

A high-nutrient, low-calorie diet enhances health in all kinds of ways. It improves the liver's ability to detoxify, enhances hormone function, helps the kidneys' blood-clearing functions, inhibits osteoporosis and improves the integrity of connective tissue (the ageing of which shows up in wrinkles). Mice fed a calorie-restricted diet look younger, friskier and leaner, are sexually active and fertile for longer and score better in cognitive tests.

How a low-calorie, high-nutrient diet works

When you eat, a by-product of toxic waste is generated in which billions of rogue electrons known as 'free radicals' wreak havoc in your body, laying the foundation for serious diseases and causing ageing of cells. The high-nutrient, low-calorie diet both limits the amount of free radicals generated *and* provides the fruits, vegetables and whole grains that are rich in anti-oxidants and neutralise the effects of free radicals (see Chapter 7 for more about antioxidants and free radicals).

Why would you want to live longer?

When people hear that there is a possibility of extending life-span beyond 120 years, they commonly react by saying, 'Ugh –

I wouldn't even want to live to 120, thanks.' They do not realise that by practising calorie restriction you can have a thirty-year-old body rather than a forty-year-old one, even if you're thirty-five, and that you may be able to add healthy, active years or even decades to your life, perhaps including a second or third career. If you are already in your forties or fifties, it is not too late to start – calorie restriction significantly extends the lifespan and healthspan of animals who do not begin it until middle age, although the earlier you start, the better.

How much should you eat?

If you currently overeat, cutting your calorie intake by around 10 to 20 per cent, but no more, should bring optimum benefits, and cutting intake by a smaller amount will still do you good when eating high-nutrient, low-calorie food. If you don't want to count calories, eat until you are only just full, then push your plate away, even if there is still something on it. You should feel neither overly hungry nor overly full. For those who do want to count calories, Roy Walford recommends an upper limit of 2,200 calories daily; the people described in this book eat around 2,000 calories on average. Remember to make allowances for your height and how active you are.

You should always eat plenty of high-nutrient foods, which will keep you healthy and satisfied but will be low in calories. If you feel low in energy, you are not eating enough of the right foods – a high-nutrient, low-calorie diet should make you feel better, not worse. Fibrous foods such as fruits, vegetables and whole grains are bulky and filling, and should leave you feeling pleasantly full without being stuffed. Studies also show that nutrient-rich foods prevent cravings.[4]

Do not crash diet. By eating a nutrient-dense diet you should lose weight slowly, steadily and permanently. Crash dieting is bad for health, rarely works and speeds up the ageing process. One fashion model has recently revealed that after she kept her weight down by living for seventeen years on a diet of cigarettes, coffee, mineral water and the occasional chocolate croissant, her hair became completely white and she had to have surgery to mend three holes in her heart.[5] Do not feel that you will necessarily become thin on a reduced calorie, nutrient-dense diet, because we are all built differently. This is not a problem – genetically obese mice have extended lifespans and much better health on a low-calorie, high-nutrient diet.

Do not substitute more exercise for fewer calories. Eating high numbers of calories and then burning them off with exercise will not bring the health benefits of calorie restriction, as you will still be creating the ageing effects of fuel use within the body. It is good to take regular exercise, but for health generally rather than as part of calorie restriction.

A note of caution: calorie restriction is not for children, who are still growing. For optimum benefits, Roy Walford recommends beginning at twenty years of age.

What should you eat?

Imagine that you live in a wholly natural environment, as the Biospherians did, rather than on a street lined with supermarkets and junk-food shops. What would you be eating? The answer is that anything you could pick or catch, such as fruits from a tree, fresh greens or the odd fish from the river, would provide you with a nutrient-rich diet. In brief, a nutrient-dense diet includes plenty of fresh fruits and vegetables, some whole grains, beneficial fats such as those found in oily fish and nuts and seeds (see Chapter 11), and sufficient protein, preferably derived from vegetables such as beans and pulses rather than from animal fats (see Chapter 9).

IN SUMMARY

A low-calorie, high-nutrient diet

- Eating a high-nutrient, low-calorie diet is the only proven and highly effective method of slowing the rate of ageing and extending lifespan.

- Eating this type of diet significantly reduces the risk of serious diseases and slows the rate of ageing.

- You can eat a moderated version of the diet and still enjoy the benefits.

- There is no need to feel deprived as eating high-nutrient foods is more satisfying than eating low-nutrient foods.

- There is no need to count calories as eating high-nutrient foods automatically means taking in less calories.

- If you are overweight, lose weight slowly and steadily for permanent weight loss by eating just 10 to 20 per cent fewer calories than you normally do.

- Aim to eat exactly what you need and no more of high-quality food.

- Bear in mind that the populations in this book all *naturally* eat high-nutrient, low-calorie diets.

7

Eat a variety of fruits and vegetables

•

I am not a vegetarian because I love animals; I am a
vegetarian because I hate plants.

A. WHITNEY BROWN, *comedian*

FRUITS AND VEGETABLES ARE THE CINDERELLAS of our diet –
crucial, delectable, but so often neglected. Yet one of the
most conspicuous things about the diets of the five
populations discussed in Part I is that they all include large
amounts of fresh fruits and vegetables. Even the men love their
juicy apples and pears, roasted red peppers, seaweed and other
fruits and vegetables (who doesn't love a runner bean they've
grown themselves?). Current anti-cancer recommendations are
that we eat a minimum of five servings of fruits and vegetables
daily; most of us have less, while the people that have been
described in Part I have up to ten servings.

Antioxidants to the rescue

Fruits and vegetables are full of all kinds of nutrients essential for your good health. The last chapter explained how calorie-restricted diets only work when the food eaten is rich in nutrients, which means including large amounts of fruits and vegetables. Plant foods contain fibre, which aids digestion – an essential part of optimum health (see Chapter 13). Most plant foods also contain at least five different vitamins and minerals that your body needs in order to perform its biochemical reactions. A healthy head of broccoli, for example, contains calcium, magnesium, phosphorus, B vitamins, beta-carotene and vitamin C.

The main reason why fruits and vegetables are such effective anti-ageing agents, however, is that they contain large amounts of antioxidants, which have the power to neutralise ageing 'free radicals' – rogue molecules that go rampaging through your body, damaging other molecules by 'oxidising' them. Your body is subjected to continual attack from free radicals; it can be likened to an apple going brown or an iron nail going rusty. Medical science now accepts that free radical damage accounts for at least 70 per cent of all disease, including arteriosclerosis, Alzheimer's disease, cataracts, arthritis, stroke, cancer and accelerated ageing.

Right now, as you breathe and when you metabolise food, your body is generating millions of free radicals, each one of which causes a chain reaction in which a million or more molecules are damaged. You can speed up the damage by taking in extra free radicals from outside the body. Pollution, drinking, smoking (one puff generates over a trillion free radicals) and eating deep-fried and burnt foods all add to the load – if you enjoy it, it probably creates free radicals.

Antioxidants are molecules that stop free radicals in their tracks and prevent them from doing damage. You make your own antioxidants in your body, but you need extra from the vitamins and minerals found in fresh fruits and vegetables (since they also need to protect themselves from free radicals). Antioxidants are such an excellent safeguard against disease that Dr Richard Cutler, Director of the US Government Anti-ageing Research Department, has said 'the amount of anti-oxidants that you maintain in your body is directly propor-tional to how long you will live'. Most people, however, do not eat nearly enough antioxidant-rich fruits and vegetables. Jean Carper, author of *Stop Ageing Now!* believes that 'much of what we call ageing is really a fruit and vegetable deficiency'.[1]

Fruits and vegetables – the true fountain of youth

Biotech companies are spending enormous sums of money searching for lucrative cures for illness and ageing, but the answer is right here in front of us on a plate. In Roy Walford's calorie-restriction tests (*see page 114*), maximum lifespan was extended significantly, but only when the diet was high in antioxidants. Antioxidants prevent free radicals from damaging the DNA in cells and wrecking cell membranes, both of which can lead to cancer; one major world-wide study has shown that eating fruits and vegetables can cut cancer risk by half.[2] Antioxidants also protect the heart by preventing the oxidation of LDL cholesterol (see Chapter 10).

Antioxidants protect tissues from 'cross-linking', a process that causes old leather suitcases, and our faces, to become worn and wrinkled. A little cross-linking is necessary to hold every-thing together, but free radicals can cause too much, leading not only to aged skin but also to stiffened arteries and damaged DNA. To test your cross-linking, put your hand flat on a table surface. Take a pinch of skin from the back of your hand and pull it upwards. If it springs back your cross-linking damage is minimal. The longer it stays raised, the more cross-linking damage you have.

How many antioxidants do you need?

Researchers at Tufts University in Boston have devised a measure for antioxidant power called ORAC, or 'oxygen radical absorbency capacity'. A good number of units to aim for is between 3,500 and 6,000 per day. Prunes are extremely high in antioxidants, and eating 10 prunes will provide 4,620 units, while 100 grams of blueberries contain 2,234 units. Other fruits and vegetables, such as cucumbers, are far lower in units, so aim for five to ten servings daily of a range of fruits and vegetables to keep your intake high. Heating destroys antioxidants, so try to eat most of your fruits and vegetables raw or lightly cooked.

ORAC Scores for Foods[3]

Food	Score per 100g (approx. 4 oz)
Prunes	5770
Raisins	2,830
Blueberries	2,234
Blackberries	2,036
Kale	1,770
Strawberries	1,536
Spinach, raw	1,210

Food	Score per 100g (approx. 4 oz)
Raspberries	1,227
Plums	949
Alfalfa sprouts	931
Spinach, steamed	909
Broccoli	888
Beetroot	841
Avocados	782
Oranges	750
Grapes, red	739
Peppers, red	731
Cherries	670
Kiwifruit	602
Beans, baked	503
Grapefruit, pink	483
Beans, kidney	460
Onions	449
Grapes, white	446
Corn	402
Aubergines	386
Cauliflower	377
Peas, frozen	364
Potatoes	313
Potatoes, sweet	301
Cabbage	298
Lettuce, leaf	262
Cantaloupe melon	252
Bananas	221
Apples	218
Tofu	213
Carrots	207
Beans, string	201

Food	Score per 100g (approx 4 oz)
Tomatoes	189
Courgettes	176
Apricots	164
Peaches	158
Squash	150
Beans, lima	136
Pears	134
Lettuce, iceberg	116
Watermelon	104
Melon, honeydew	97
Celery	61
Cucumber	54

Which antioxidants?

Most antioxidants come from vitamins and minerals, which are found in greatest abundance in fruits and vegetables, but also in nuts, seeds, whole grains and animal products (although you should avoid eating too much meat – see Chapter 9). So far, a hundred antioxidants have been identified in various types of food, with the best-known ones being vitamins C and E, beta-carotene (the precursor of vitamin A), selenium and zinc. You need to consume a wide spectrum of antioxidants, as they work in concert – for example, vitamin C rejuvenates spent vitamin E. Therefore aim to eat a wide range of fruits, vegetables and whole foods. It is also a good idea to take a supplement containing several antioxidants including these top five.

THE TOP FIVE ANTIOXIDANTS

Vitamin C

Food sources Most raw fruits and vegetables, especially red peppers, citrus fruits, strawberries, papaya, berries, broccoli and green salad leaves.

Vitamin E

Food sources Wheat germ, olive oil, avocados, nuts and seeds, and cold-pressed nut and seed oils.

Beta-carotene/vitamin A

Food sources of beta-carotene Red and yellow fruits and vegetables such as carrots, sweet potato, squash, pumpkin and apricots; dark green leafy vegetables such as spinach and watercress.

Food sources of vitamin A Oily fish, cod liver oil and liver.

Selenium

Food sources Brazil nuts (these are very rich in selenium; two straight from the shell will give you all you need for the day), garlic, mushrooms, asparagus, sesame seeds, sunflower seeds, yeast, whole grains, organ meats, meats and seafood.

Zinc

Food sources Oysters, shellfish, organ meats, whole grains, pumpkin seeds, sesame seeds, okra, green leafy vegetables and peas.

Eat a range of colours

Where you find colour and flavour in a fruit or vegetable, you will also find the most antioxidants (notice how cooking removes colour and flavour, as well as killing antioxidants). The reds, yellows and oranges of tomatoes, squashes and carrots, for example, are due to the presence of beta-carotene. Foods that are very rich in colour, such as blueberries, raspberries and red grapes, are particularly rich in powerful antioxidants called proanthocyanidins. Since antioxidants work together, it is important to eat foods in a wide range of colours during the day. The dishes of the long-lived people discussed earlier, such as the sweet-potato-loving Okinawans or the tomato-eating Mediterraneans, are often very colourful when laid out on a plate.

When preparing meals, aim to use foods in at least five different colours, including, for example, orange carrots, red and yellow peppers, green spinach, purple cabbage, blackberries and raspberries. For a quick and delicious multicoloured antioxidant lunch, try the Sweet Potato Salad recipe (*see page 106*), which uses orange, dark green, light green, purple, red and black.

Enjoy your antioxidants

Make your salads appealing with olives, herbs and lightly steamed vegetables such as beans or asparagus, and always include a delicious dressing with extra-virgin olive oil and garlic (both of which are full of antioxidants). Add a small knob of butter or lemon and olive oil to lightly steamed greens for flavour, or steam-fry them in garlic, ginger and soy sauce. In order to reach your quota of five to ten servings daily, aim to eat a large helping of vegetables twice a day, plus one or two pieces of fruit as a snack. After a while, your eating habits and taste buds will adapt, and you may find that you start to really miss fruits and vegetables if you don't eat them for a day or so.

IN SUMMARY

Antioxidants versus free radicals

- Aim to eat five to ten servings of fruits and vegetables daily.

- Try to eat foods of several different colours at each meal, as antioxidants work in concert.

- Eat raw or lightly steamed fruits and vegetables so as to retain antioxidants.

- Take an antioxidant supplement containing vitamins A, C and E, and selenium and zinc.

- Try to avoid accessing free radicals from pollution, smoking and barbecued or deep-fried foods.

chapter

8

More raw food

•

THE LONG-LIVED PEOPLE I described in Part I like to pick their food raw and eat it just as it is. After all, why cook it when this just removes flavour and wastes time and fuel? Fresh apricots, leafy, herby salads, raw garlic and grapes eaten straight off the vine – raw foods are versatile, convenient and delicious, and they still have most of their nutrients left in them when they arrive at the table, because they have not been destroyed by cooking.

When the people featured in this book do cook their food, they do so for only a short time, so that there is a minimal loss of nutrients. Vegetables are often steamed for just a few minutes or quickly boiled in a very small amount of water. The Hunzakuts heat their chapattis for only a minute or two, so they get most of the benefits of the vitamin E-rich wheatgerm, while Okinawans stir-fry their vegetables for a minimum amount of time, keeping them fresh and crisp. The inclusion of raw or lightly cooked food in the diets of these people is an important factor in their remarkable health and longevity. It is also an aspect of their diets that is easy and pleasurable for you to emulate.

Don't cook!

Man is the only species that cooks food. We discovered how to make our own fire a mere 400,000 years ago, after several million years of evolving specifically to eat raw foods such as fruits, vegetables, roots, shoots, seeds, and raw meat and fish. Raw foods contain within them everything that is necessary not only to sustain life but also to keep us in a state of absolute health.

The produce you see at your greengrocer's or growing in a vegetable patch is an incredible natural dispensary of immune-boosting, cancer-inhibiting, life-lengthening substances, more complex and effective in their chemical structure than any man-made drug ever invented. The more you heat and process your plant foods, the more you destroy these substances.

Raw foods provide enzymes, the 'spark plugs' that initiate every one of the millions of biochemical reactions in your body that keep you alive. You make your own enzymes from the vitamins and minerals you eat, but not enough to keep you in a state of optimum health, so you also need to get them from food. Enzyme production drops with age, which means that the amount of enzymes you have is a measure of how fast you are ageing. Living organisms such as fruits, vegetables, nuts and seeds are rich in enzymes that keep them healthy and fight off toxic substances, and when you eat these foods, you get the benefits. Up to 100 per cent of these enzymes, however, are killed by heating.

Raw foods are highest in vitamins, minerals and anti-oxidants, including a very important anti-ageing substance, superoxide dismutase, which is lost with cooking. As much as 75 per cent of the vitamin C content of a cabbage is lost in boiling, and 50 per cent of vitamin E is lost in frying or baking. Cooking plant foods in water causes minerals to leach out and be lost. Cooking protein foods also denatures the amino acids we need so that they are of less use to us, and even harmful.

The fibre in raw food has the most effective broom-like quality for sweeping out the intestines, ensuring that food does not putrefy in the gut. There are different kinds of fibre, each with its own use, and if you eat plenty of salads and fruits you will get them all in ample quantities. Between them these various types of fibre aid peristalsis (the movement of faeces through the colon), make you feel fuller for longer, regulate blood sugar levels, dilute harmful substances, encourage friendly bacteria, remove carcinogens such as excess bile acids, and cause less fat to be absorbed by the body.

'Miracle' cures from raw food

Raw food appears to have an amazing ability to heal people of all kinds of ailments, from headaches to cancer. Max Gerson, a medical student in Berlin at the turn of the twentieth century, cured himself of severe migraines with a salt-free, mostly raw food diet. When he tried out the same diet on his patients, he found that it was an unqualified success not just for those with migraines but also for those with 'incurable' tuberculosis, and the diet was adopted by some of the greatest TB experts of his day. Gradually, it transpired that the diet worked for nearly all illnesses, and also reversed signs of ageing.

When Gerson gave cancer patients high levels of nutrients from raw fruits and vegetable juices, he found that their bodies could frequently regain balance and heal themselves, even when the cancer was supposedly terminal. Cell activity was restored to normal, and toxins that had built up around cells drained out of the body, removing the cause of the disease and thus healing the body.

Raw foods to make you youthful

People changing to raw food diets have reported that, as a result of the improved circulation of nutrients and the removal of toxins from cells, their skin looks tighter and is much less puffy, their eyes become clearer, and any grey hair they have starts to grow back dark. Collagen is responsible for the elasticity of our skin, and it is kept in production by the vitamin C that comes in a raw food diet. Cellulite has also been found to disappear on a raw food diet, partly because raw foods help to eliminate the toxins that are linked with cellulite.

Studies show that raw foods can help you to lose weight without suffering any of the agonies and failures of going on a diet.[1] Raw foods expert Dr John Douglass has said: 'For many years I struggled with obesity and was frustrated in treating patients because nothing ever seemed to work . . . Then I discovered the potential of uncooked foods and found that the more uncooked foods patients used, the less they wanted to eat. These foods are more satisfying for patients and they lose weight on them.'[2]

How to eat raw foods

Dedicated raw-foodists eat 80 to 90 per cent of their food raw. If you find this difficult, aim to eat two-thirds or more of your food raw, which still leaves room for going out to dinner and enjoying plenty of warm soups and stews in the winter. If you must cook your vegetables, steam them lightly or gently stir-fry them for just a few minutes so as to lose a minimum of nutrients. At the least, try to eat three pieces of fruit, a handful of nuts and seeds, and a salad every day.

Raw food is quick and easy to prepare – instead of worrying about recipe ideas you just chop up whatever vegetables you have and drizzle salad dressing over them. Raw food does not have to mean 'rabbit food' – it also includes nuts, olives, yoghurt, olive oil, and sushi, to name just a few. If you are having a pre-dinner drink, instead of crisps try eating chopped carrots, cauliflower and broccoli dipped in hummus or guacamole. You can also make fruit salads and treat yourself to some papaya or pineapple, which are both particularly rich in enzymes.

IN SUMMARY

Raw foods

- Raw foods offer higher levels of nutrients, including vitamins, minerals and fibre, than cooked foods.

- Raw foods contain all the enzymes necessary for their digestion; cooking kills up to 100 per cent of the enzymes.

- Raw foods may be useful in curing cancer and other illnesses associated with ageing.

- A diet high in raw foods is very effective for losing weight without going hungry.

- Try to eat around two-thirds of your food raw in the form of fruits, salads, raw vegetables, nuts and seeds, and sushi.

Less meat, more vegetable protein

It always seems to me that man was not born to be a carnivore.

ALBERT EINSTEIN

THE PEOPLE WHO ARE THE FOCUS OF THIS BOOK illustrate clearly how you must emphasise vegetables, rather than meat, in your diet if you want to a live for a long time. It isn't that these people don't love meat; it's just that it is not readily available to them, so it is eaten only as a special treat around once a week, or in small amounts to flavour vegetable-based dishes. Moreover, their animals are very different from the fattened, overgrown animals pumped full of antibiotics and sold in our supermarkets today. They keep lean and wholesome by roaming the mountainsides and pastures grazing on organic, nutrient-rich grasses.

Dispelling the myth

It is a myth that humans need to eat animal protein in order to gain sufficient meat and muscle. The average adult male gorilla weighs 800 pounds and thrives very happily on a vegan diet of vegetables, fruits and nuts. True, we are only relatives of the gorilla, but the latest research in sports nutrition shows that our top athletes not only build sufficient muscle, but also do best in terms of endurance and stamina when following a vegetarian diet. Animal protein does help us grow, but it gets us in the end by laying the foundations for disease. When laboratory animals are fed on animal protein, they mature and grow more quickly than those on a vegetarian diet, but they also die earlier.[1]

You do need to eat protein, however. Without it, you would be a slushy, watery creature, not resembling a human being at all. When you digest protein it is broken down into amino acids, which are the building blocks of your body (*see page 145*). However, the way for you to maintain good health is to eat the right kind of protein – that is, *vegetable protein* rather than animal protein (*see page 144* for good sources of vegetable protein). The Oxford Vegetarian Study has recently found that cancer mortality is 39 per cent lower among vegetarians than it is among meat-eaters.[2] Another study showed that on average, vegetarians develop degenerative diseases ten years later than meat eaters do, and that they visit the doctor half as often.[3]

A system suited to a vegetarian diet

Your colon is long, like that of a grass-eating horse or cow, rather than short like that of a flesh-eating lion. When the putrefying, bacteria-riddled products of meat digestion reach your colon, they linger there for days or weeks, smearing themselves stickily over your colon wall and impacting themselves in any cavities they can find. They then break down into carcinogenic substances; some of these are reabsorbed by your body and others stay there until some plant fibre comes along and, hopefully, takes them out with it.

Your teeth are also best suited to a vegetarian diet. You chew from side to side with your large, flat molars, which are shaped for grinding grains and grasses, and any meat you eat has to be tenderised first by cooking, marinating or being bashed with a hammer. It is then broken down to some extent by the hydrochloric acid in your stomach, but this is much weaker than that of true carnivores. Cats, for example, secrete ten times more hydrochloric acid than we do.

Animal protein as a toxin

Dr Colin T. Campbell of Cornell University and co-chairman of the World Cancer Research Fund was raised on a dairy farm and milked cows from the age of five to twenty-one. He now believes that 'animal protein is one of the most toxic nutrients there is'. His view is based on his findings from the China Project, which was led by him and is the biggest study of population and diet there has ever been. The study data show clearly that mainly vegetarian Chinese from rural areas have far lower rates of heart disease, stroke, osteoporosis, diabetes and cancer than urban Chinese eating a meat-based diet. The data also reveal that the rural Chinese have only *6 per cent* of the amount of heart disease that North Americans have.

Dr Campbell believes that the main reason for these findings is that animal fats, which are high in saturated fats, raise levels of harmful LDL cholesterol in the blood, which is associated with higher rates of degenerative diseases (see Chapter 10 for more about cholesterol). Plant foods, on the other hand, reduce LDL cholesterol levels. Dr Campbell hypothesises that 80 to 90 per cent of Western diseases such as cancer, heart disease and diabetes could be prevented before the age of around ninety years if we substituted plant protein such as pulses and beans for animal protein.[4] Of course, the rural Chinese also get the other benefits of eating vegetables rather than meat, such as high levels of antioxidants.

Avoiding cancer with a meat-free diet

The populations described earlier all have exceptionally low levels of cancer, and one important reason for this is their low meat intake. Dr Campbell has said 'in my view, no chemical carcinogen is nearly so important in causing human cancer as animal protein'.[5]

The link between meat intake and cancer is well established. Back in 1976, John Morgan, the president of Riverside Meat Packers in the US, attempted to counteract the damage done to the meat industry by publicity over a very strong link between meat-eating populations and colon cancer.[6] He said, 'Beef is the backbone of the American diet and it always has been. To think that meat of all things causes cancer is ridiculous.' Six years later he died of colon cancer.[7]

The China Project has shown that the Chinese have only one-third the amount of colon cancer that Americans have, which its authors believe is due to the comparatively low consumption of meat in China. Other studies back up these findings. In 1990, Dr Walter Willet found in a study of 88,000 women aged thirty-four to fifty-nine that those eating red meat daily had over twice the risk of getting colon cancer than those eating it less than once a month. He said, 'if you step back and look at the data, the optimum amount of red meat you eat should be zero'.[8]

Research shows that there is a close link between eating animal fats and hormonal cancers such as breast and prostate cancer.[9] Dr Robert Kradjian, breast surgeon for thirty years and author of *Save Yourself From Breast Cancer*, says, 'breast cancer is essentially a dietary disease, just as lung cancer is essentially a smoking-related disease. If you want to avoid breast cancer, then learn to live like the billions of women on this Earth who will avoid the disease. Eat as the women in protected countries do – a diet high in protective vegetables, fruits, and fibre – a plant-based diet.'

The worst types of meat

Of all types of meat, processed meats such as hot dogs, bacon and salami appear to be the worst culprits.[10] Hot dogs and other cured meats are treated with nitrites and nitrates, which form highly carcinogenic nitrosamines in the stomach (these are also found, in much higher levels, in cigarette smoke).

There is some confusion here because most of the nitrates in our diet come from vegetables that have been treated with nitrate-containing fertilisers; yet vegetarians suffer from up to 40 per cent less cancer than meat eaters do. Scientists do not yet understand all the factors at work, but until they do it's best to play safe by avoiding cured meats and eating organic nitrate-free vegetables if possible. If you really want to eat cured meats from time to time, combine them with fruits and vegetables, especially tomatoes, as the Campodimelani do, as the antioxidants in them have a protective effect.[11]

Cooking methods to avoid

Cooking meat on a high heat, for example by frying, grilling and barbecuing, creates carcinogenic HCAs, which are also found in tobacco smoke.[12] These develop in the cooked meat even where it isn't browned, so you cannot scrape them off.

If you want to eat cooked meat, oven roasting and baking produce fewer HCAs, and boiling, stewing or poaching generate hardly any. Interestingly, tests by Dr John Weisburger show that if soya is added to meat it blocks the formation of HCAs during cooking. Also, antioxidants help neutralise the formation of HCAs, so if you do eat meat, have it with a salad. Fish is a better option than meat as it produces only around a fifth of the amount of HCAs, even when cooked at high temperatures.

Chicken and fish: the differences

Do not confuse chicken with fish. Chicken is a little leaner than fatty red meat, but it is still full of saturated fat, as you will know if you have ever stuck a skewer into the side of a roast chicken and watched the fat oozing out. Our battery chickens are also fed with growth-promoting antibiotics that may be hazardous to health. Eggs are high in cholesterol but do not seem to raise cholesterol levels in the body, so it is probably fine to eat them now and again, especially if they are from free-range chickens fed on seeds,.

Fish is undoubtedly the best source of non-vegetable protein as it contains beneficial essential fatty acids, and you should eat oily fish regularly (see Chapter 11). The Okinawans, Bama people, Campodimelani and Symiots all enjoy fish twice a week or more; none of them are regular chicken eaters.

Leave cow's milk to the calves

There are those who believe the day may come when you have to go on safari to see a cow. Unfortunately for cows, this is not the case at the moment. The cows you see decorating fields along the motorway are not representative of their kind. Today, a typical dairy cow in the developed world spends her whole life pregnant (a very unsatisfactory way to be, especially as she never gets to be with her offspring), trapped for months in a concrete stall with barely room to move, possibly on a slatted metal floor, being milked regularly by a noisy machine. She and her millions of peers are sick, unhappy, highly medicated animals, raised purely in order to produce as much milk as possible at the minimum cost.

Why does this happen? So that we can drink regular supplies of a substance which is very good for the health of and designed exclusively for *calves*. Cow's milk has a very specific protein, mineral and essential fatty acid content, which is not suitable for human consumption. After weaning age, many people lose the enzyme lactase, which is needed to digest the lactose in milk.

Research shows that cow's milk can cause child-onset diabetes, anaemia in babies, asthma, excess mucus, rheumatoid arthritis, indigestion, oestrogen dominance and athero-sclerosis, among other illnesses.[13] Breast-feeding women with colicky babies frequently find that their child's health problems disappear when they stop drinking milk. No other species would dream of continuing to drink milk after being weaned. Who trained us to adopt this bizarre behaviour – nature, or the dairy industry?

We are frequently told that we should eat dairy products so as to avoid osteoporosis. Yet most Africans and Asians, and the people studied in this book, drink very little milk and they also have extremely low rates of osteoporosis. On the other hand, those countries where most dairy products are eaten, such as the United Kingdom, United States, Finland and Sweden, have the highest rates of the disease.[14] This is most likely to be because heat-treated milk and cheese are acid-forming in the body. Our bodies cannot function in an acidic environment, so they borrow alkaline calcium and magnesium from our bones to buffer the acid. Many vegetables, however, contain both calcium and magnesium, and are alkaline-forming in the body.

What about iron?

Plants should be able to provide you with all the nutrients you need, including calcium and iron. After all, where did the cow get the iron in the first place if not from eating grass? Iron deficiency rates for the meat-eating North Americans and British are relatively high, while subjects of the China Project and the people studied in this book have good iron status. One reason for this is that vegetarians tend to consume more vitamin C, which is needed for the proper absorption of iron.

Vitamins B12 and D

There are just two nutrients that you can get from meat but cannot get from plant foods: vitamin B12 and vitamin D. Vitamin D is manufactured by the action of sunlight on skin, but strict vegetarians may need to take vitamin D supplements, particularly if they don't live in a sunny climate. The best food source of vitamin D is oily fish.

Vitamin B12 is obtained from meat, fish or tofu, and it is also made by 'friendly' bacteria in the gut. It is needed only in small amounts, and deficiency is rare. However, it is an important nutrient, and it is wise to make sure you have enough. If you are a vegan or have been a strict vegetarian for some time, it is a good idea to check your levels of vitamin B12 and to take supplements if you are deficient (see Chapter 18 for supplements). Nursing mothers on a vegetarian diet should take particular care to supplement B12.

The best sources of protein

The protein sources that are healthiest for you are plant foods and fish. Good sources of vegetable protein are nuts and seeds, beans such as kidney beans and soya beans, and lentils. The populations described earlier all regularly eat these foods, as well as fish. All plant foods contain some protein, even lemons. Spinach is 49 per cent protein, almost as much as steak, which is 52 per cent protein. A balanced vegan diet that includes a range of green vegetables, pulses, nuts, seeds and grains should provide you with all the protein and other nutrients you need. The chart below provides information on protein amounts in different foods.

Sources of protein

Food	Protein (grams)
100 g (4 oz) spinach	48
90 g (3½ oz) chicken	32.8
120 g (4½ oz) soya beans	28.6
150 g (5 oz) cottage cheese	25
75 g (3 oz) fish	20.3

Food	Protein (grams)
200 g (7 oz) lentils	17.9
100 g (4 oz) quinoa	16
120 g (4½ oz) kidney beans	15.4
125 g (4½ oz) millet	8.4
240 ml (8 fl oz) whole milk	8
120 g (4½ oz) yoghurt	7.9
25 g (1 oz) walnuts or almonds	7
1 egg	6.1
100 g (4 oz) pasta	6
200 g (7 oz) white rice	6
100 g (4 oz) oatmeal	6
200 g (7 oz) brown rice	4.5
1 slice bread	2

The eight essential amino acids

You must get enough amino acids from your food. There are twenty-five amino acids in different types of protein, eight of which are 'essential' (nine for children), meaning that they are essential for life but you cannot make them in the body. Certain types of protein are *complete proteins*, meaning that they contain all eight essential amino acids. These are found in meat, fish, eggs, dairy products and some vegetables.

Since animal products are not an ideal food source it is preferable to obtain your daily amino acids from vegetables, grains, nuts, seeds or fish. Either eat individual vegetables that contain all eight essential amino acids, or eat plant foods containing a combination of proteins during the day, mixing and matching (*see lists below*). This way you are likely to get all eight amino acids within twelve hours.

VEGETABLES CONTAINING ALL EIGHT ESSENTIAL AMINO ACIDS

Soya
Hemp
Quinoa
Avocado
Millet
Spirulina (available in supplement form)
Chlorella (available in supplement form)

Note that meat, dairy products and fish contain all eight essential amino acids

PLANT COMBINATIONS CONTAINING ALL EIGHT ESSENTIAL AMINO ACIDS

Whole grains (e.g. brown rice, brown bread, chapatti) + lentils (e.g. dhal)
Whole grains + nuts
Whole grains + beans (e.g. kidney beans)
Beans + nuts or seeds
Hummus + brown bread

How much protein do you need?

The World Health Organisation recommends that we eat 35 grams protein daily; other sources recommend 44 grams daily for men and 36 grams daily for women. The people discussed in Part I tend to eat around 50 grams of protein daily (some more, some less), most of which is vegetable protein. We certainly need a lot less protein than we eat: the average Briton eats around 128 grams daily and the average American 151 grams. Different amounts suit different people, so experiment with what makes you feel best. Some groups, such as infants, pregnant and lactating mothers, and growing teenagers, need more protein, but not necessarily much more. US nutritionist Dr Michael Colgan, adviser to Sylvester Stallone and many Olympic athletes, states that if you are a body builder trying to gain your maximum muscle potential you only need 2.8 grams of extra protein a day – the equivalent of half an egg.

Animal protein and you

If you like meat and cheese, then have it. There is no point in eating food that you find unappetising. The key is to change the ratios around, so that vegetables and grains form the main part of the meal, and meat is used more for flavour than bulk – your meal will contain fewer calories this way. Trim off the excess fat from meat, and stew the meat, skimming the fat off the top of the water. Less can be more, and by limiting the amount of meat you eat you will really appreciate it – you will also be justifying the expense of buying really good, organic lean cuts.

IN SUMMARY

Animal protein

- Eat meat in small amounts, infrequently – try not to have it every day.

- Do not fry or barbecue meat: stew it instead and scrape away the fat during cooking.

- Trim the fat off meat.

- Eat organic meat when possible.

- Use meat to flavour vegetable dishes rather than the other way around; aim for a vegetable to meat ratio of 4:1.

- Choose fish rather than meat.

- Choose mainly vegetable protein foods.

- Make sure you get all eight essential amino acids.

chapter

10

Keep your blood vessels young

•

CARDIOVASCULAR DISEASE, namely heart disease and stroke, is the number one cause of death in the US and the UK. Atherosclerosis, the clogging of the arteries that causes cardiovascular disease by blocking the passage of nutrients to the heart and other vital organs, is commonly accepted as an inevitable part of ageing. Yet for the people that have been described in Part I, it is virtually unknown.

In Okinawa, there are 80 per cent fewer heart attacks than in North America, while cardiologists studying the Hunzakuts found no evidence of cardiovascular disease in a sample of men in their nineties. These people stay young and add years to their lives by keeping their arteries young and elastic, and so can you.

High cholesterol levels from eating fats have traditionally been blamed for atherosclerosis. However, it is not just cholesterol on its own that causes the problem. Studies show that people eating fat-free, low-cholesterol diets sometimes fare even worse than those on high-cholesterol diets in terms of heart attack and stroke rates. The Campodimelani, who are very fond of olive oil, have been found to have cholesterol levels as low as those of infants, and Eskimos, who live on a high-cholesterol diet, have some of the lowest heart attack rates in the world. Before you race out to buy a large, fatty leg of lamb from the butcher, read on to discover exactly what you should and shouldn't eat in order to keep your arteries clear.

Cholesterol – fatty sausages in your veins

'In 1953, as I completed the final stages of my first autopsy as a medical student, I saw something I'll never forget,' writes Dr Charles R. Attwood. 'While sectioning the heart of a nine-year-old girl who had died suddenly and unexpectedly of meningitis, I found yellow deposits within one of her coronary arteries. "Take a good look," the pathology professor said, "you'll probably never see this again during your entire career." The yellow deposits proved to be cholesterol . . . Today, 42 years later, nearly 50 million American children have abnormally high blood cholesterol levels. . . By the age of 12, two-thirds of all children, like the little girl on my autopsy table, have the beginning stages of coronary disease, which eventually accounts for a third of all adult deaths'.[1]

Cholesterol is a waxy, fat-like substance found in plants and animals, including us. We need it to transport fat-soluble anti-oxidants to cells and repair fatty cell membranes, and for this reason we manufacture some cholesterol ourselves, although we only need very little. Both 'good' and 'bad' cholesterol can be found in our bloodstreams. Cholesterol cannot travel through the blood on its own so it has to get a lift with a spherical body called a lipoprotein. 'Bad' cholesterol is transported from the liver to the arteries by Low Density Lipoproteins (LDLs), while 'good' cholesterol is transported from the arteries back to the liver by High Density Lipoproteins (HDLs).

In order to keep your veins clear of cholesterol, therefore, you want to keep your HDL cholesterol level high (above 50 mg/dL) and your LDL cholesterol level as low as possible (below 100 mg/dL). In fact, a high overall cholesterol level with a good ratio of HDL to LDL cholesterol is probably preferable to a low overall cholesterol level (150 or below) with a bad ratio. The heart-disease-free people described earlier tend to have fairly low cholesterol levels with a good ratio. The Okinawan elders, for example, have an average cholesterol level of around 170, with an overall cholesterol to HDL ratio of around 3.3:1.[2]

The role of cholesterol

LDL cholesterol is taken to the arteries for the very good reason that the arteries are sometimes in need of repair, and LDL cholesterol serves as a useful sticking plaster. The device is not foolproof, unfortunately, because while it may temporarily stave off death from leaking blood vessels, it can cause death by clogging them instead. The blood vessels nearest to the heart are the most susceptible to wear and tear because of the pressure of the blood being pumped by.

When a blood vessel develops a small tear, or lesion, LDL cholesterol comes along and sticks itself over the tear. It then gets oxidised by passing free radicals and 'plaque' is formed. Doctors performing post mortems know plaque to be long, yellow, fatty, sausage-like formations in the veins (imagine pulling melted mozzarella cheese out of a straw). These may block the passage of blood to the heart or brain, causing a heart attack or stroke.

Maintaining healthy cholesterol levels

To maintain healthy cholesterol levels try to do the following:

1. Eat plenty of plant foods – the antioxidants will help prevent the oxidation of cholesterol, while the fibre in vegetables and whole grains will assist in the removal of excess cholesterol from the body.

2. Avoid saturated fats and hydrogenated fats found in animal foods and processed foods respectively, as these raise LDL cholesterol levels (see Chapter 11 for more about the fats you need to avoid).

3. Obtain good fats by eating oily fish, nuts and seeds. These raise HDL levels and lower LDL levels (see also Chapter 11).

4. Avoid refined carbohydrates, such as white flour and sugar, as these raise blood sugar levels, which in turn brings about a harmful cholesterol ratio (see Chapter 12 for more on refined carbohydrates).

5. Take regular exercise, as this has been found to improve cholesterol levels.

Vitamin C to avoid 'scurvy of the arteries'

According to two-time Nobel laureate Linus Pauling, PhD., the best way to avoid lesions from forming in your arteries in the first place is by ensuring that you have a high vitamin C intake. Vitamin C is required to make collagen, which is essential for artery health and elasticity. Pauling noted that it is only species that do not make their own vitamin C, such as humans and guinea pigs, which tend to suffer from atherosclerosis. He felt that the role of vitamin C is so crucial in preventing athero-sclerosis that he renamed the disease 'scurvy of the arteries', after the vitamin C deficiency disease.

Pauling and his colleague Mathias Rath found that the equivalent of the recommended daily allowance (RDA) of vitamin C (60 grams) offered almost no protection against arterial damage, whereas much higher doses can reverse arterial damage in humans.[3] He recommended a minimum of 3 grams of vitamin C daily; he himself took up to 18 grams daily, and lived an active life until the age of ninety-three. To protect your arteries, take a supplement and eat vitamin C-rich foods such as green leafy vegetables, blackcurrants, mango, papaya, green peppers and oranges.

Hypertension – a reversible condition

The greater the force with which the blood is pumped around the blood vessels, the greater the wear and tear on the blood vessel walls, which is why hypertension, or high blood pressure, is a major cause of heart attack and stroke. Some of the many symptoms of hypertension include dizziness, lethargy, headaches, insomnia, restlessness, difficulty in breathing and emotional instability.

It is widely believed that hypertension is an inevitable consequence of increasing age, yet fifty million Americans under the age of sixty-five suffer from hypertension. The long-lived people described in this book, on the other hand, are notable for their low blood pressure levels, even in old age. One study has shown that making simple changes to the diet can be as effective as taking hypertension drugs.[4]

Is your blood pressure healthy?

You can ask your doctor to measure your blood pressure.
It is measured on two levels. The higher level is 'systolic',
which is the pressure when the heart is contracting, and
the lower level is 'diastolic', which is the pressure when
the heart is resting between pulses.

Good	90/60 to 125/85
OK	126/86 to 135/89
Borderline	136/90 to 145/95
Dangerous	146/96 and above

To lower your blood pressure

You can avoid high blood pressure by adopting the following
diet and lifestyle practices.

1. **Reduce stress** This has been found to be very effective for
   lowering blood pressure, whereas high stress raises it.[5] See
   Chapter 20 for how to reduce stress.

2. **Take exercise** The heart is a muscle, and needs exercise just
   like all the other muscles in your body. When the heart is
   strong, it can pump more blood with each beat, so that fewer
   beats are needed to get the blood moving and blood pressure
   is lowered. See Chapter 29 for more about exercise.

3. **Do not overeat** Obesity and the consumption of too many
   saturated and hydrogenated fats from meat and processed
   foods are both linked with hypertension.[6]

4. **Avoid excess alcohol** This can be a main cause of high blood pressure, although moderate amounts of red wine are preventive.[7]

5. **Drink green tea** This contains less caffeine than coffee, which can cause high blood pressure.[8]

6. **Avoid refined carbohydrates**, such as white bread and sugar. These raise insulin levels, which in turn causes high blood pressure. Eating whole grains has the opposite effect.[9] See Chapter 12 for more about which carbohydrates to eat.

7. **Limit salt consumption** Too much salt causes the muscles to put extra pressure on the arteries, which raises blood pressure.

8. **Avoid smoking** This constricts the arteries, which increases blood pressure.

9. **Take vitamin E** This is found in olive oil and oily fish, but is best obtained from supplements. It has been found to be almost four times more effective than aspirin for lowering hypertension by thinning the blood, without having side-effects.[10]

10. **Increase your intake of calcium, magnesium and potassium**, from fruits and vegetables. These minerals aid blood vessel health; there is a particularly strong link between magnesium deficiency and heart attack risk.[11]

11. **Eat antioxidant-rich fruits and vegetables**, especially garlic and onions. These reduce blood pressure, so make them a regular part of your diet.[12]

Homocysteine – the real culprit?

In 1969, an eight-year-old child who had died of a stroke, and a two-month-old baby, were found during post mortem to have severe atherosclerosis. Heart researcher Dr Kilmer S. McCully discovered that both children had normal cholesterol levels, but abnormally high levels of a substance called homocysteine in their blood. McCully was certain that it was the homocysteine that had caused these bizarre cases of premature ageing. To test his theory, he injected rabbits with homocysteine, and sure enough they developed arterial plaque within three to eight weeks.

McCully's conclusions about homocysteine were published in the *American Journal of Pathology*. It is only recently, however, that people have started to sit up and take notice of homocysteine. In 1995, the *Journal of the American Medical Association* concluded that homocysteine represents a strong independent risk for heart disease, and current research shows that homocysteine levels are forty times more predictive of heart disease than cholesterol levels.[13]

What is homocysteine?

Homocysteine is a toxic amino acid that is produced during the metabolism of protein, especially red meat, fish, cottage cheese and peanuts. If there are not enough of the B vitamins B6, folic acid and B12 in the diet to process the homocysteine, it can build up to dangerous levels in the blood. The homocysteine then oxidises any LDL cholesterol around, which causes plaque formation, and it also makes the artery walls less elastic and helps form blood clots.[14] Where there is high cholesterol, there is also likely to be high homocysteine, as both are caused by eating a diet high in animal protein and low in plant foods.

Homocysteine-promoting foods

Foods that can lead to homocysteine build-up are, in descending order: cottage cheese, fish, meat, poultry, roasted peanuts, sesame seeds and lentils. Smoking also raises homocysteine levels. The diets of some long-lived populations do include fish, seeds and lentils; however, they also eat foods that are high in B vitamins, so they avoid excess homocysteine.

Make sure your diet contains enough vitamin B6, folic acid and vitamin B12. Good sources of vitamin B6 are whole grains, sweet potatoes, baked potatoes with their skins, tuna and salmon; folic acid is found in green vegetables, and vitamin B12 can be obtained from fish and soya products.

IN SUMMARY

Keeping your blood vessels young

- Keep your cholesterol ratio healthy and avoid the oxidation of LDL cholesterol using the tips given in this chapter.

- Protect your arteries from wear and tear with vitamin C.

- Avoid high blood pressure following the above advice.

- Keep homocysteine levels to a minimum by ensuring adequate intake of B vitamins.

Eat the right fats

•

THERE ARE FATS, AND THEN THERE ARE FATS. Some kill, others heal. A common thread in the diets of the long-lived populations I have described is an absence of killing fats and an abundance of healing fats, while in the typical Western diet it is the other way around.

Long-lived populations eat essential fats from nuts, seeds and fish, which are essential for health and have many healing properties. They also consume monounsaturated fats, mainly from olive oil, which are not essential but are very good for you. Western populations, on the other hand, tend to eat saturated fats from meat and cheese, which encourage obesity and diseases of ageing, and altered fats, the most sinister types of fat of them all. These come from heated polyunsaturated oils and are found in most processed foods, such as margarine, biscuits and cereals. They are hazardous to health, yet surprisingly few people know about them, and profitable businesses rely on them (perhaps it is *because* profitable businesses rely on them that few people know about their dangers). If you care about your health, you *must* understand which fats you should be including in your diet, and which ones you should be avoiding.

The destruction of polyunsaturated fats

Today's vegetable oils are so unlike food that they may as well be used as car fuel. In fact, they are – one Cheshire company has found a way to recycle oil used by a poppadom manufacturer into a green alternative fuel called 'e-diesel', while a man from Manchester currently runs his Volvo Estate on old chip-pan oil. What has happened to our oil?

Originally, many European villages and country estates had manually operated presses with which local people made their own wonderful life-giving nut and seed oils. These oils were volatile, because the two kinds of essential fat in them, omega 3 fats and omega 6 fats, react easily to light and heat. This is precisely what makes them so useful to our bodies, as they cause many essential biochemical reactions in our cells. However, it also means that they go rancid quickly and start to generate ageing free radicals (see Chapter 7 for more about these). Back in the days of manual oil presses, the oil was delivered fresh every few days in small bottles, and was used up before it had a chance to go bad.

The cheap polyunsaturated oils sold in supermarkets today are heated to very high temperatures, refined and even bleached to give them a longer shelf life.[1] Their chemical structure is altered in such a way that they cannot be used properly by our bodies, and are thought to cause many degenerative diseases such as cancer and cardiovascular disease.

The steep rise in heart disease in the last century corresponded with the increased use of cheap cooking oils, despite manufacturers' claims that these are good for heart health. These oils *would* be good for heart health, if only they had not been destroyed by processing. Beware of any supermarket oil you see other than cold-pressed extra-virgin olive oil, because it has been processed in this way, and beware of the oils hidden in products such as mayonnaise or canned food kept in oil.

Hydrogenated fats and trans-fats – the dangerous altered fats

If you know what's good for you, you will go into your kitchen now and throw out everything containing 'hydrogenated vegetable oils', 'partially hydrogenated vegetable oils' and 'vegetable fats'. Most biscuits, almost all cereals, most chocolate, cakes, crackers, margarine, frozen ready meals and ice cream are made with these damaging, unnatural products. Their harmful effects on health are now so well known that the manufacturers have to include them on the ingredients lists for their products, even if they claim at the same time that their products are 'healthy'. These altered fats are silent but deadly killers. They have an unnatural molecular structure that sabotages our cell structure.

Polyunsaturated oils

When polyunsaturated oils are heated to high temperatures, the hydrogen atoms within their molecules flip across to the wrong sides of the molecules. The molecules become twisted and rigid, which makes the oil stable so that it can be stored for a long time. However, when the molecules get into our bodies, we accidentally use them to build cell membranes, and the cell membranes also become rigid, whereas they should be flexible. Proper cell function can no longer happen and, over the years, ageing and disease of cells occurs. When you look at the metal tub of cooking oil in a fish and chip shop, you are looking at millions of molecules of these deadly 'trans-fats'.

Hydrogenated fats

Hydrogenated fats are a type of altered fat that is created by adding hydrogen atoms to the polyunsaturated fat molecules to make them straight, packable and similar to saturated fats (*see page 162*). They are solid or semi-solid at room temperature, which makes them useful for maintaining shelf life and giving that satisfying texture to 'foods' such as chewy biscuits, chocolate, margarine and ice cream.

'Partially hydrogenated' vegetable oils have been put through a similar process to become trans-fats. If you want to eat products such as ice cream and biscuits sometimes, read the labels carefully, because you can get higher-quality brands made without these dangerous altered fats that taste just as good, if not better. Porridge oats are one of the few cereals you can buy in a supermarket that do not contain altered fats.

The effects of altered fats

You won't die from eating one chip or a bowl of ice cream, but after years of eating these and other products containing altered fats, your bodily foundations start to become shaky and vulnerable to collapse. Altered fats can also damage the DNA in our cells, which means they can harm our genes, which we then pass down to our children. Trans-fats and hydrogenated fats also contribute to heart disease by promoting blood clotting and raising LDL cholesterol levels.[2] These altered fats cannot be digested or metabolised properly, and the body needs to call on its extra reserves of nutrients to process them, which depletes the vitamins and minerals we need to ward off illness.

Trans-fats are prohibited in baby foods. What does this tell you about them? They can, however, still find their way into babies through their mothers, during pregnancy and breast feeding. According to Udo Erasmus, author of *Fats that Heal, Fats that Kill*, altered fats have many harmful effects on cell membranes, brain development, the cardiovascular system, the liver and the immune systems of foetuses and children.

Saturated fats – the bad fats

Saturated fats, or 'hard fats' (solid at room temperature), are found in animal products such as meat, dairy products and eggs. These fats are the white, greasy substance you find in your roasting pan after the gravy has cooled, and in your blood after you have eaten them.

Saturated fats are not as bad as altered fats, because the body recognises them as natural and is able to process them; it is better to use butter than margarine for this reason. Our bodies need some saturated fats and manufacture their own from carbohydrates, but too many saturated fats cause health problems such as diseases of fatty degeneration and hormone-related cancers (see Chapter 9, animal protein).

Monounsaturated fats – the good fats

Monounsaturated fats such as the extra-virgin olive oil that is used so liberally in the Symiot, Campodimelani and other

Mediterranean diets are good for health. Olive oil helps with membrane development and cell formation, improves cholesterol levels, and encourages bile secretion, which improves the digestion and excretion of fats.

The monounsaturated fats in olive oil are stable and therefore useful for cooking, although it is best to keep olive oil at low temperatures as it does contain around 7 per cent polyunsaturated fats. Avocados are another good source of monounsaturated fats, so include both olive oil and avocados in your salads. Avocado oil has recently been introduced onto the market and makes an excellent salad dressing.

Canola oil, popular in America and also used in Okinawa, contains 54 per cent monounsaturated acids and is thought to be safer than most cooking oils. However, it also contains some polyunsaturated oils, which can become damaged during the manufacturing process and in cooking. The Okinawans seem to thrive perfectly well on canola oil, but it is probably second best to extra-virgin olive oil, especially when heated.

Essential fats – the fats you MUST have

Essential fatty acids (EFAs) are so-called because they are absolutely essential for the good health of all our cells and organs and cannot be manufactured by the body, so that they have to be obtained from the diet (*see page 164*). EFAs keep away 'diseases of ageing' such as heart disease and cancer, as well as many other ailments ranging from depression and PMS to eczema, according to a mounting body of evidence.

One type of essential fat, omega 3 fats, improves heart health by helping to transport cholesterol from the blood, lowering blood pressure and preventing blood from clotting. Oily fish is high in omega 3 fats, which is one reason why fish eaters such as the Eskimos and the people discussed in this book have very low heart disease rates. EFAs also decrease tumour formation and the metastasis of cancer, and can even kill cancer cells.[3]

There are so many other benefits from EFAs that it is hard to know where to start. EFAs are anti-inflammatory, and so help to prevent asthma and rheumatoid arthritis. They keep cell membranes flexible, which allows them to let toxins out and nutrients in, and keeps your skin soft and supple. They are essential for brain and nervous system function, and have been found to be very effective for improving mental health (see Chapter 16). They improve metabolism, and so can help with weight loss, despite being relatively high in calories.

How to get your essential fats

There are two types of EFA: omega 3 (alpha linolenic acid) and omega 6 (linoleic acid). They are provided by polyunsaturated acids in their fresh, unspoiled state. Oily fish is the best source of omega 3 fats, while fresh nuts and seeds straight from the shell provide mainly omega 6 fats (see list below).

We need both types of EFA in the right ratio, as too much of one or the other can cause health problems. A perfectly balanced body needs about 4 per cent of total calories (about a tablespoon daily) from omega 6 fats and 2 per cent (one to two teaspoons daily) from omega 3 fats. However, the typical Western diet contains around twenty times more omega 6 fats than omega 3 fats, which is very unbalanced. Too many omega 6 fats are implicated in blood clotting, inflammatory disease and some cancers.[4]

To compensate for this, you should emphasise omega 3 fats in your diet, at least for a while so as to regain balance. Try to eat oily fish such as mackerel, herring and organic salmon around twice a week. These contain the end products of omega

3, which our bodies so desperately need: eicosapentaenoic acid (EPA) and docosahexaenoic acid (DHA).

You can also obtain EPA and DHA from fish-oil capsules; make sure you buy a good brand from fish from clean waters, and one that is regularly checked for freshness, and throw them out if they start to smell fishy. DHA can also be obtained from the yolks of eggs from free-range chickens fed on an omega 3-rich diet. With the exception of the Hunzakuts, all the populations discussed in this book eat fish regularly.

Omega 3 fats also come from plant sources such as flax, walnuts, soya, dark green leafy vegetables and hemp seeds, which are a staple of the Bama diet. However, when we get EFAs from plant sources, we have to metabolise EPA and DHA ourselves, which many of us cannot do efficiently, so fish is more useful. For those who dislike fish (or like them enough not to want to eat them!), hemp oil is a good source of both omega 3 and omega 6; it can be bought in health-food shops. Eating nuts and seeds straight from the shell or as fresh as possible will also provide some essential fats, mainly omega 6 fats.

Listed below are the best food sources of omega 3 and omega 6 fats. If you buy oils, they should come in dark, refrigerated bottles from health-food suppliers; they should *not* be common supermarket oils. Supplements containing both kinds of EFA are also available; consult your health practitioner or local health store. Note: fish oil capsules may not be suitable for infants.

OMEGA 3 SOURCES

- *Oily fish* such as mackerel, herring, salmon, sardines and tuna (buy organic salmon so as to avoid high levels of toxins).

- *Flax oil* (linseed oil) contains four times as much omega 3 as omega 6. It is therefore useful for short-term use to correct imbalances.

OMEGA 6 SOURCES

- *Sunflower seeds* and their oil.

- *Sesame seeds* and their oil.

- *Corn* and its oil.

- *Wheatgerm* and its oil.

- *Pumpkin seeds* and their oil.

- *Safflower seeds* and their oil.

OMEGA 6 AND OMEGA 3

- *Soya*.

- *Hemp* – contains three times as much omega 6 as omega 3.

- *Walnuts* – fresh and preferably straight from the shell to avoid rancidity.

- *Organic free-range eggs from seed-fed chickens* These may have a 1:1 ratio of the two fats, whereas battery eggs can have nineteen times more omega 6.

- *Seaweed* – contains small quantities of EFAs.

- *Shellfish* – contain small quantities of EFAs.

- *Dark green leafy vegetables* such as spinach, parsley or broccoli – contain small quantities of EFAs.

- *Most unprocessed whole plant foods* – contain small quantities of EFAs.

Bear in mind that all the essential fatty acids in the world will do you no good if you cannot process them, and if your diet lacks the necessary nutrients to do this, they may even do you harm. In order to convert EFAs into their desired end-products, you need a range of vitamins and minerals to metabolise them, as well as fat-soluble antioxidants such as vitamin E and vitamin A to prevent them from going rancid in the body. Alcohol, saturated fats, tobacco and fried foods all block EFA metabolism, and should be avoided or severely restricted in the diet.

For a more detailed description of EFAs and why you need them, read Udo Erasmus's *Fats that Heal, Fats that Kill*.

IN SUMMARY

Fats

- Essential fats (EFAs) are essential for the correct functioning of every cell, tissue, organ and gland in your body.

- Most people in the UK and the US are deficient in essential fats, especially omega 3 fats.

- Monounsaturated fats, found in olive oil, are the good fats and are safest for cooking.

- Saturated fats, from meat and dairy products, are bad fats.

- Altered fats from supermarket oils and processed foods are highly damaging to your body cells and functions, and are implicated in causing cancer and heart disease.

- Ensure adequate intake of vitamins and minerals to aid EFA metabolism.

- Follow the example of the people I've described in the first part of this book: eat fish, whole grains, nuts and seeds, and fresh fruits and vegetables.

12

Eat whole grains

●

> As you know, in white bread the germ, with its wonderful
> health-giving properties, is extracted, and put into chicken-
> food. As a result the human race is becoming enfeebled,
> while hens grow larger and stronger with every generation.
>
> Davey Warbeck in *The Pursuit of Love*.
>
> NANCY MITFORD, British writer

SHOULD WE BE EATING CARBOHYDRATES OR NOT? The answer
lies in the fact that refined carbohydrates such as white
bread and white rice are stripped of nutrients and cause
disease and weight gain; while unrefined carbohydrates like
whole wheat and brown rice promote health.

The traditional diets of the long-lived people discussed
earlier include whole grains and avoid refined carbohydrates.
While carbohydrates can raise blood sugar levels, which can
have all kinds of health implications, these people do not eat
the high-meat diets currently fashionable with those in the
West seeking to lose weight and stabilise blood sugar. Their

vegetable- and whole-grain-based diets protect them from diabetes, cancer and heart disease, which are correlated with high blood levels of insulin and glucose.

The rise of white bread

In the old days, before there was an epidemic of degenerative disease, fresh home-made bread was baked daily, using just wholewheat flour, water and a little yeast. This is how bread is still made by the Hunzakuts, Campodimelani and Symiots, and it is doubtless responsible at least in part for their good health. The germ of a whole grain such as wheat is the part used to grow a new plant, so it is packed with many life-giving substances including folic acid, B vitamins, iron, zinc, magnesium, potassium, selenium, vitamin E and phytochemicals. Whole grains also provide fibre, which is essential for good digestion (see Chapter 13).

A modern supermarket loaf, mass produced and spongy in its plastic bag, conveniently never seeming to go hard or mouldy, is made quite differently. The pesticide-treated wheat first goes to the flour mill, where the germ and husk of the grain are removed, taking with them the all-important fibre and 87 per cent of the nutrients. Just four nutrients are put back – iron and three synthetic B vitamins.

The finished loaf is given a squashy texture and super-quick rising ability by adding extra gluten and yeast, both of which are known to cause gastrointestinal disorders. The loaf may be made with such joys as hydrogenated vegetable oils, sugar, preservatives, and 'improvers' to keep it soft and 'fresh'. Artificial colouring may be added to make it brown.

Carbohydrate addiction

If you crave a pizza, chocolate eclair or crumpets for tea, the chances are that these are the very things you should be avoiding. White flour products are fast burning – that is, they are broken down very quickly in the body, and too much of their end product, sugar, is released into your bloodstream at once.

Too much blood sugar is harmful, so the pancreas panics and lets out too much insulin to get rid of it, causing blood sugar levels to fall too low. Some time after eating the pizza or eclair, you feel a dip in energy, often experienced mid-afternoon as a feeling of fatigue and a craving for something sweet. You reach for the biscuit tin, and the whole cycle begins again. These swings in blood sugar levels are called hypoglycaemia, and a great many of us suffer from it.

Eventually, after years of abuse, the cells in the body get fat, start behaving differently, and stop answering so readily to the insulin's knock. They are now insulin resistant, and the result is that there is too much glucose circulating in the blood, unable to get to the cells.

People who are insulin resistant continually feel tired, as the cells have less of the energy they normally get from glucose. Some of the glucose gets converted to fat, and the growing epidemic of obesity in the UK, the US and other Western countries has been strongly linked to a diet high in refined carbohydrates. Obesity is a good predictor of shortened lifespan (how many obese eighty-year-olds have you met?).

Insulin resistance also causes too much insulin to circulate in the blood, which eventually leads to adult-onset (Type II) diabetes, a disease that has been linked to a diet high in refined carbohydrates.[1] Type II diabetes was once thought of as a disease of ageing, but in the UK, where we each eat 75 kilos of white flour per year, there is a growing epidemic, and even children are starting to develop it.[2]

Sugar ages you

Anyone with diabetes or insulin resistance can expect to have signs of accelerated ageing. Excess insulin causes your genetic material, DNA, to turn over more quickly, which speeds up the ageing process. Studies have also shown that insulin stimulates the growth of cancer cells.[3] As diabetics are aware, hyper-insulinism is the most reliable predictor of heart disease, because insulin raises levels of 'bad' LDL and 'very bad' VLDL cholesterol.[4]

Sugar is sticky, and it likes to stick to, or form complexes with, the proteins in your body that make up most of your tissues and also your genetic material. This process is called glycation, or glycosylation, and the unsavoury result is a tangle of cross-linked structures called Advanced Glycosylation End-products, otherwise known as AGEs. When food is fried or browned, the same process occurs, only much more quickly – in other words, it is as though you were being slowly cooked. The brain tissue of Alzheimer's patients contains clumps of AGEs, whereas that of healthy people does not.[5]

Slow down ageing with slow-burning foods

The Glycaemic Index (GI) is a measure of how much certain foods raise blood sugar levels, gauged against pure glucose, which tops the score at 100. By eating slow-burning unrefined carbohydrates that are low on the GI, you can prevent and perhaps even reverse those 'diseases of ageing' caused by an over-zealous insulin response, including cancer.[6] Most whole grains, vegetables, beans and pulses are low on the GI; fruits are also fine to eat as they contain fructose rather than glucose, which is absorbed differently by the body.

As you can see from the lists below, some foods, such as baked potatoes and French bread, are so high on the GI that you might almost as well inject them straight into your veins. Eating these foods in smallish quantities with low GI foods such as vegetable protein or salad will lower the overall glycaemic load of the meal.

Brown rice and wholemeal bread are strange aberrations, since they are as high on the GI as their refined counterparts, but they have higher nutrient value and more fibre. Mixed whole grain bread is lower on the GI than ordinary brown bread, so choose chewy-looking loaves with mixed grains for slower digestion. Avoid eating too much of anything at one sitting, as this will raise blood sugar levels too high.

Animal protein is the slowest burning food of all as it contains no carbohydrates, and this is the reason for the current popularity of high-protein diets such as the Atkins diet. They can be useful for getting rid of carbohydrate addiction, but should only be used for short periods of time. Animal products bring other health problems with them, such as colon cancer, so choose fish rather than meat and dairy products. Another way to reduce insulin response is to cut down on salt. A little wine with a meal may also be beneficial, as studies have shown that it can stop the formation of AGEs.[7]

Glycaemic Index of common foods

High Glycaemic Index foods (70–100) – restrict

Baked potatoes, mashed potatoes (up to 100)

Baguette (95)

Sugar, honey, sweets, cakes, biscuits

Cooked carrots

White bread, crumpets

Wholemeal bread

White rice, brown rice

Sugary drinks

Most commercial breakfast cereals such as corn flakes

Dried fruits and bananas

Medium Glycaemic Index foods (40–70) – include

Boiled potatoes, sweetcorn, raw carrot, sweet potato

Pasta

Barley bread, rye bread

Mixed wholegrain bread and seed breads

Basmati rice

Porridge oats, bran cereals, muesli

Pitta bread

Grapes, mango, figs, kiwi fruit

Low Glycaemic Index foods (0–40) – enjoy

Beans and pulses

Nuts and seeds

Apples, peaches, oranges, plums

Most vegetables including broccoli, cauliflower, lettuce, mushrooms, leeks, tomatoes

Oily fish

Dairy products (keep to small quantities for other reasons)

70 per cent cocoa chocolate (as above)

Other problems with refined carbohydrates

Refined carbohydrates are also hazardous to health in other ways. For example, when white rice was first introduced to Asia it brought an epidemic of the deficiency disease beriberi. Research published in the *Lancet* has also shown that women who eat the most food made from white flour (such as white bread, biscuits and pies) have the highest incidence of breast cancer.[8]

Whole grains contain a large range of vitamins and minerals that are crucial for health, such as zinc, magnesium, vitamin E, chromium, potassium and iron. Unlike refined carbohydrates, whole grains also contain fibre, which keeps your colon healthy. The B vitamins found in whole grains provide the enzymes you need to digest carbohydrates, fats, and proteins; one sign of B vitamin deficiency is dry skin and hair, because essential fatty acids are not being properly absorbed. When you eat refined grains such as white rice or white flour, your body has to borrow from its reserves of B vitamins in order to digest them and, over a period of time, diseases of vitamin B defiency can start to occur. These include heart disease from excess homocysteine build-up, mental disorders, and diseases of the brain and nervous system (such as beriberi).

Sensitivity to grains

Many people have problems digesting grains, particularly wheat, with a quarter of the UK population thought to be wheat intolerant. This may be because for two million years of human evolution there were no grains in the diet – grains were strictly for the birds. Bread is a staple of the Campodimelani,

Symiot and Hunzakut diets, however, and they don't seem to suffer. This may be because their wheat is not treated with pesticides and other chemicals, and their bread is also lower than ours in gluten, which irritates the gut. Eating bread in relaxed surroundings, and chewing it to perfection, also helps with digestion. If you are sensitive to wheat or other grains, you may find that eating them in small quantities does not cause problems.

Guide to grains

There is a huge variety of grains available apart from whole wheat. By experimenting with some of the grains described below, you should be able to find a few that suit you.

BROWN RICE

Contains magnesium, iron, B vitamins and fibre; gluten-free. Try brown risotto rice in a mushroom risotto for a rich nutty flavour, or Japanese brown rice noodles with garlic and soy sauce. Also try Chinese red rice, another whole grain form of rice that looks beautiful and has much more flavour than white rice.

PORRIDGE OATS

Easily digestible, improve cholesterol ratio and regulate blood sugar levels. Use in porridge with nuts and a little honey, or to make oat cakes and biscuits.

HEMP

Contains all eight essential amino acids, B vitamins, potassium, magnesium, calcium and iron; gluten-free. Hemp is also an excellent source of essential fatty acids and ready-made GLA, and contains omega 3 and omega 6 fats in the right balance for long-term health. It is a staple of the Bama diet. Hemp pasta has an excellent texture and flavour and goes well with pasta sauces.

MILLET

Easily digested, contains all eight essential amino acids, helps collagen formation; gluten free. The only alkaline-forming grain. Try millet flours, breads and pastas, available from health-food shops.

QUINOA

Easily digested, contains all eight essential amino acids, calcium and iron; gluten free. Good with tomato sauce and in salads containing garlic.

SPELT

A more digestible, ancient cousin of modern wheat that is higher in protein, fibre, and B vitamins and lower in gluten. Try spelt pastas and breads, which have an excellent flavour and texture and are available in health-food shops.

BARLEY

Full of B vitamins, calcium and potassium. Good in soups.

BUCKWHEAT

Lowers blood pressure, contains the anti-cancer agent vitamin B17 and is a good source of fibre, protein, B vitamins and minerals. Soba noodles made from buckwheat are available from health-food and oriental shops; soba noodle soup is popular in Japan as a hangover cure.

CORN

Contains some antioxidants which are increased by cooking, and is gluten free. Eat on the cob, as polenta or in corn bread.

KAMUT

A rich source of iron and B vitamins, and is low in gluten. Kamut pasta, which is available from health-food shops, has a good texture and a delicious nutty flavour.

AMARANTH

Rich in protein, fibre, vitamins and minerals; gluten free. Used by the Bama people; available from health-food shops in the form of pastas and flour products, which have a nutty, malty taste.

IN SUMMARY

Good and bad carbohydrates

- Whole grains contain many essential nutrients, whereas refined grains have been stripped of them.

- Many 'diseases of ageing' are diseases of excess insulin, caused by a diet high in sugars and refined carbohydrates.

- These diseases can be prevented and perhaps even reversed with the right diet.

- Avoid refined carbohydrates such as white breads, cakes, and biscuits.

- Mix medium or high GI foods with low GI foods for an overall low glycaemic load.

- Avoid eating too much at one sitting to prevent a high glycaemic load.

- Eat grains in moderate quantities and chew well for good digestion.

13

Mind your stools

•

Death sits in the bowels and bad digestion is the root of all evil.

HIPPOCRATES, ancient Greek 'Father of Medicine', 400 BC

FORGET PALM-READING – if you really want to know how long you're going to live, take a look at your stools. Your faeces should be large, almost odourless, moist, well-formed, buoyant and easily evacuated, and you should feel afterwards that the motion has been complete. You should also be going once a day at the absolute minimum, and ideally twice or even three times, once after each meal. You are constipated if you go less than once a day, have bowel movements that involve strain, or produce hard stools or stools that sink.

Problems with the digestion

Constipation is thought to be at the heart – or bottom – of a great many diseases of Western civilisation. The people described in Part I do not get constipated, because they have diets and lifestyles that promote the easy passage of stools and make sure that nutrients get to their organs to keep them in fine working order. Many of these people cite good digestion as a reason for their remarkable health and longevity.

When you are constipated, faeces linger in your colon, so that the bloodstream reabsorbs the poisonous substances that were supposed to be expelled and carries them to tissues and organs all around the body, causing a wide range of ailments and more serious diseases. Bad breath, excess weight, body odour, mouth ulcers, headaches and mental illness can all be caused by a sluggish bowel.

Your skin is a good indicator of the way your bowel is working – little bumps and pimples, oily areas or dry, flaky ones are reliable signs that all is not well with your digestion. More obvious constipation-related illnesses include colon cancer, diverticulitis, appendicitis, piles, fistula, colitis, ulcers and biliousness. Gastroenterologist Dr Anthony Bassler wrote in 1933, after a 25-year study of over 5,000 cases, 'Every physician should realise that the intestinal toxaemias are the most important primary and contributing causes of many disorders and diseases of the human body.'

Improving your digestion

If you do not take steps to rectify minor problems such as constipation or bad skin, you are headed away from health and towards more serious (although common) conditions associated with a modern diet. The best thing you can do for yourself if you want to look good, enjoy life and slow the ageing process is to adopt eating habits that will keep your digestion working well. By improving your digestion you can shed excess weight, gain more energy, and look and feel younger.

Eat easily digested foods

We have Stone Age colons, but we eat a twenty-first century diet, and the two are incompatible. The diet eaten by the world's longest lived populations, which emphasises fruits, vegetables and whole grains, and avoids refined foods and saturated fats, is best suited to our digestive systems in all ways. Include as many of such foods as possible in your diet. In addition, olive oil will help the passage of stools through your gastrointestinal tract, and it is a good idea to also include a little live yoghurt in your diet, as the 'friendly' bacterial cultures in it aid digestion and keep your intestinal tract healthy.

Smell your food and look at it

The people described earlier love cooking and eating, and they make and eat their food with care. When you eat, start by sitting down and breathing in the delicious aroma of your salmon noodles, or roast vegetables with herbs or whatever it is you have chosen to have. Look at the beautiful colour combinations of the foods that are (hopefully) arranged on your plate – oranges, whites, reds and greens, along with tasteful garnishes of herbs such as coriander or parsley. This process should activate your saliva, digestive juices, enzymes and digestive hormones, which will greatly assist the process of digestion.

Chew your food

Put the first forkful in your mouth, and start chewing. Taste the delicious flavours as they flood through your mouth. Try to chew each mouthful twenty times or more – Mahatma Gandhi, the great chewing expert (and Indian leader), once said that you should 'eat your drinks and drink your food'. Chewing helps to produce saliva and reduces the surface area of the food so that the enzymes can get to work on it. It also sends a message to the stomach to get the hydrochloric acid going for protein digestion. Chewing can help you to lose weight – it ensures that the message that the stomach is full gets to the 'satiety centre' in the brain so that you don't overeat.

Relax

Always take the time to relax and enjoy your meals, since this is an excellent way to aid digestion. Sit down when you eat, and don't forget to breathe. If possible, avoid eating at the computer or at the wheel of your car (I once read about a man who was arrested at Christmas for negotiating a roundabout using his elbows to turn the steering wheel while he demolished a turkey carcass).

Try to minimise stress, which reduces the all-important digestive enzymes and hydrochloric acid and depresses the immune system, which in turn is needed to maintain a healthy gut. After eating, avoid getting up for fifteen minutes. Breathe in and feel your breath entering your abdominal area, relaxing the stomach as you do so. This may help with any anxiety-related digestive problems.

Graze, don't gorge

The Okinawans eat until they are only *almost* full; other long-lived populations do not stuff themselves, as they have limited supplies. Gudrun Jonsson, author of *Gut Reaction*, recommends eating no more at one sitting than can be held in your two cupped hands, which corresponds to the amount of room in the stomach. Eating until you are stuffed puts a burden on the gut. It also undermines the benefits of the healthy food you are eating since undigested food, no matter how nutritious it is before you ingest it, can turn toxic. Eat until you are only just full, and have a snack later if you get hungry.

Eat away from sleep

Sleep and food do not make good bed partners. You cannot digest food properly and sleep at the same time. Eat a satisfying breakfast, a moderate lunch and a light supper, and try to leave four hours between dinner and going to bed. Try to leave at least half an hour after getting up before eating breakfast to give your digestive system a chance to wake up. Many of the long-lived villagers described earlier work in the fields for an hour or two before breakfast.

Drink water

All of the populations described in this book drink fresh water, traditionally from local rivers. As well as helping to detoxify the body (see Chapter 14), water aids the passage of food and bulks out the faeces so that they can be squeezed out more easily. Try to drink at least eight good-sized glasses of water daily, away from your food. Do not use water to wash down food – drink it away from meals, so as not to dilute your digestive juices.

Exercise regularly

The muscles lining the colon cannot squeeze faeces out properly unless they are kept working with regular exercise. If you have ever found that your constipation was relieved by going for a good long walk, you will have experienced this. Walk briskly for twenty minutes a day or take some other form of exercise.

Squat, don't sit

When you move your bowels, try placing your feet on a low stool in front of you. When our bowels were first designed several hundred thousand years ago, toilets had not yet been invented and the two are not quite compatible. The bowel has a slight kink near the exit, and faeces can get stuck in this kink if we go to the lavatory in the sitting position. The Hunzakuts squat in a yogic position over their lavatories (which strengthens their thigh muscles at the same time).

Eat fibre – the intestinal broom

Fibre acts like an intestinal broom, bulking out the faeces and creating stools that glide effortlessly through and out of the digestive tract. Studies have shown that traditional societies that eat high-fibre foods have almost zero rates of the illnesses linked to a low-fibre diet, such as diabetes, appendicitis, colon cancer, heart disease, diverticulitis, piles and constipation.[1]

The typical Western diet contains only around 10 to 15 grams of fibre; we should be eating at least twice that, according to National Cancer Institute recommendations. The SAD (Standard American Diet) is almost guaranteed to clog up the system, as saturated fats and refined carbohydrates are sticky and mucus forming. No wonder people become overweight on the SAD. Since fibrous foods, on the other hand, move through the system efficiently, you can eat more of them and still lose weight.

The best sources of fibre are fruits, vegetables and whole

grains, as eaten by the long-lived people discussed in Part I. Wheat bran, which your doctor may have recommended for constipation, is the worst source of fibre, as it scratches and irritates the intestines. Beware also of 'high-fibre' breakfast cereals, which are often processed, full of sugar, have to be eaten with milk and are usually made with grains that have been dry cooked, which makes them almost indigestible. Psyllium husks and linseeds soaked overnight are extremely useful fibre supplements. I find that figs, pineapple and papaya are all also excellent for getting things moving.

Combine your foods the Hay way

In the early 1900s, a doctor called William Howard Hay found himself, at the age of forty, seriously overweight and suffering from a chronic kidney condition, high blood pressure and an enlarged heart. He was told by physicians that he would almost certainly never regain his health. However, Dr Hay proved them wrong by correctly identifying the source of his problems – faulty digestion. 'Death begins in the colon,' he announced, and set to work devising a new way of eating. Within a relatively short time Dr Hay had lost fifty pounds and eradicated his health problems, as well as those of many of his patients whom he put on the diet.

The basic principle of the Hay diet is to improve the digestion by eating certain foods separately; most crucially, starches (such as bread and potatoes) and proteins (especially the richest proteins, animal products). Just as you cannot brush your teeth while combing your hair, so the body cannot break down proteins at the same time as it breaks down starch. By combining foods correctly, the body can work much more efficiently to absorb the nutrients it is given, and use spare energy for detoxification and metabolism.

Practitioners of food combining claim that patients who are overweight, underweight, arthritic, diabetic, insomniac, anxious, depressed, hypertensive, hypoglycaemic or constipated, or suffering from headaches, Crohn's disease, heart disease, Raynaud's disease, colitis, indigestion, migraine, premenstrual tension or irritable bowel syndrome, (just for a start) find their energy returning and their symptoms disappearing when they combine their foods properly.

Dr Hay made the important observation that people with an acidic system – the familiar grouchy, irritable, paunchy types who go out for steak and chips at lunchtime and follow it up with a handful of indigestion tablets – tend to suffer more from illness than other people. A slightly alkaline system is the ideal environment for good health. Cancer cells thrive in an acid environment, but dislike an alkaline one.

Dr Hay recommended eating mainly fruits and vegetables, which keep the system alkaline (meat and carbohydrates create acid conditions). According to Dr Hay, when carbohydrates are eaten, these should be whole grains rather than refined carbohydrates, for better digestion.

Long-lived peoples eat a moderated form of the Hay diet. They sometimes combine vegetable proteins with starches, but they do not eat much meat, so do not commit the ultimate Hay crime of combining rich animal protein with starches. They also eat an alkaline-forming diet based on fruits and vegetables, and they eat whole grains rather than refined carbohydrates.

There is more to the Hay diet than the basic outline given here, and if you want to give it a serious try you should consult a nutritionist or one of the available books on the subject, which also contain useful recipe ideas.

Cleanse your system first

Good digestion is essential for health and longevity, and if you pay attention to your digestive system now you are sure to reap the benefits both immediately and in the long term. To get the maximum benefits, you should really consider cleansing your system first. The best diet in the world cannot help you if your system is clogged with stuck toxic matter. The next chapter explains how you can give your digestive system an invaluable kick-start that will leave you feeling years younger and inspire you to change your eating habits forever.

IN SUMMARY

Good digestion

- Good digestion is essential for good health; constipation leads to illness.

- Avoid constipation with a diet emphasising fibrous foods such as fruits, vegetables and whole grains.

- The way you eat your food can be as important as what you eat.

- Exercise regularly to keep the muscles lining your digestive tract working.

- Combining foods the Hay way can help digestion.

- Cleanse your system regularly (see Chapter 14).

14

Detox, don't botox

•

You take rotten care of your body, paying it little attention at all until you suspect something's going wrong with it. You do virtually nothing in the way of preventive maintenance . . . then you fill it with toxins and poisons and the most absurd substances posing as food. And still it runs for you, this marvellous engine; still it chugs along, bravely pushing on in the face of this onslaught. It's horrible.

NEALE DONALD WALSCH, *Conversations with God*

THE BEST ANTI-AGEING DOCTOR in town is your own body. Nature is capable of many extraordinary feats, and the human body has a powerful ability to heal itself, *when given the right conditions*. Unfortunately, modern living means that for most of us, those conditions are just not there. Every time you breathe in car exhausts, feel stressed, consume sugar, take medicine, use shampoo or eat a packet of crisps you add to your body's toxic load.

The poor overworked liver tries frantically to disarm all the millions of free-radical-producing toxins and expel them through the skin, urine, mouth, breast milk, mucus, bowel or any other outlet it can find; this is what sometimes causes spots, mouth ulcers, bad breath, a coated tongue and boils to appear. Our livers were never designed to have such a full in-tray, and because most people are nutritionally deficient, the body also lacks the materials needed for detoxification. The toxins end up getting into the bloodstream, which dumps them around the body, in fat and connective tissue, to be sorted out 'another time'.

Your body – a disease time bomb

This process turns us into disease time bombs, ticking away for years or decades until eventually, inevitably, something has to give. Some of the greatest physicians in history have firmly believed that disease – *all* disease – is the result of a body becoming clogged by toxicity. 'There is but one disease,' royal surgeon Sir Arbuthnot Lane once said, 'and that is deficient drainage.'

Even once disease has set in, the body will still do everything it can to throw out the toxins and repair the damage. We sneeze, cough, have a fever, bleed, spit or form pus – all signs that the natural healing mechanisms are working away. We then, often mistakenly, take medicines that bring down the fever or stop the coughing, so that the symptoms disappear, leaving the poisons – to which the medicines' residues have now been added – inside us. If we continue in this direction, the body goes in a downwards spiral towards irreversible disease, ageing and finally death.

Avoiding poisoning your system

The long-lived people described earlier avoid toxins from cigarettes, processed foods, meat, pesticides and alcohol. They also tend to live in rural mountainous or coastal areas, where there is very little pollution. Any toxins they do acquire can be eliminated through their nutritious, fibrous diets. They take plenty of exercise, which gives them an opportunity to sweat out their toxins and boost circulation. The Hunzakuts traditionally fasted during the lean weeks between winter and spring before the new harvest came in, which is thought to be one reason for their extreme good health. Below I discuss the incredible and speedy effects that fasting can have on you.

You too can create balance in your body and expel as many toxins as are taken in, so that you remove the conditions for degenerative disease. By giving your body a good spring clean in the ways outlined in this chapter, you can cleanse your blood and tissues and give your body time to sort out its 'in-tray'. So don't botox, detox – it's the best way to take the years off.

Fasting may save your life

Hippocrates, the ancient Greek 'Father of Medicine', fasted many of his patients, claiming that 'when one feeds a sick person, one feeds only the sickness', and Greek philosophers such as Pythagoras recommended fasting for a clear mind. Jesus famously fasted for forty days at a time; and Mahatma Gandhi was another great fan of fasting.

At the beginning of the last century, a teenage boy called Herbert Shelton observed that whenever the animals on his parents' farm were sick, they would refuse to eat for a few days, and would then recover. This tendency of sick animals to fast when they were ill was familiar to farmers, who called it the 'nature cure'. Shelton himself experimented with a short fast which, he found, made him feel markedly rejuvenated. He started to read everything he could get his hands on about fasting and nutrition.

Shelton eventually opened his own health school in San Antonio, Texas, where he supervised water-only fasts for people who came to him with a range of illnesses, many of them serious and supposedly incurable. Their ailments included elevated cholesterol, high blood pressure, oedema, rheumatoid arthritis, cysts, benign tumours, appendicitis, digestive problems, obesity, alcoholism, heart disease, backache, headache, kidney stones, insomnia, prostatitis, hernia, fibroids, eczema, gallstones, sterility, mental illness, arthritis, ulcerative colitis, multiple sclerosis; some of them supposedly needed surgery, or were about to die. With just a few exceptions, people with every kind of illness appear to have benefited from Shelton's care, and many of them 'miraculously' recovered complete health.

The people who fasted looked and felt younger, and had clear eyes and few skin complaints, even in later age. In his bestselling book *Fasting Can Save Your Life*, Shelton wrote, 'some of the most remarkable examples of rejuvenation I have witnessed have been in men and women past sixty'. During his lifetime, around 35,000 people came to Shelton and took part in a fasting programme.

Water-only fasting

A water-only fast is thought to be the most rapid and efficient way to detoxify, although some health practitioners believe that juice fasting (*see below*) is preferable. Fasting is not a cure in itself; rather, it gives the body the chance it so desperately needs to cleanse itself and begin healing.

For the first three days of a fast, toxins are expelled and the blood is cleansed. Enzymes that are no longer needed by the stomach go to the bloodstream and start destroying pathogens, diseased cells and toxins. At around five days, healing and rebuilding of the immune system begins. From ten days on, disease may begin to be reversed and prevented. Serious illnesses and other conditions may begin to disappear at around thirty days. Some time after this, the body signals that it is time to end the fast with a return of appetite, sweet breath, a clear tongue and a feeling of enormous well-being.

Most people do not like the idea of water-only fasts – going without any food at all is an alien concept to modern Westerners. There is currently nowhere in the UK where you can go for a water-only fast, although there are fasting centres abroad (*see* Resources, *page 284*, for contact details). If you decide you would like to try a long fast (more than three days), you must make sure you do it under supervision, especially if you are on medication.

Fasting is safe for nearly all people, and is mainly contra-indicated under certain conditions such as pregnancy and lactation, advanced cancer and diabetes. You can get the benefits of a long fast by doing short water-only fasts of two or three days at home and repeating them every few months. If you do decide to do a short water-only fast, make sure you consult a health practitioner or read a book on the subject (*Thorson's Principles of Fasting* by Leon Chaitow is useful). Some brief guidelines for fasting are outlined below.

BASIC PROCEDURE FOR A SHORT WATER-ONLY FAST

● Fast for no more than two to three days at a time.

● Prepare yourself for the fast by eating only raw fruits and vegetables for three days beforehand.

● Avoid coffee and tea before fasting so as to lessen the effects of caffeine withdrawal.

● During the fast, relax as much as possible, at home.

● Drink two to three litres of distilled water each day – you will put your health at risk if you do not drink enough.

● Break the fast *carefully and gently* with a glass of apple and carrot juice, or an apple chewed very thoroughly. Follow with a glass of diluted juice every two hours and one or two pieces of fruit or raw vegetables in the evening. Slowly incorporate other foods over the next few days.

● Eat live sugar-free yoghurt after the fast to replace the friendly bacteria that have been lost.

● Take light exercise before and after the fast, and during it if you have the strength. Exercise is an essential part of the detoxification process as it boosts circulation and lymphatic drainage.

Juice fasts

If you want to fast but think a water-only fast is not for you, you can opt for a modified version of the fast using fruit and vegetable juices rather than water for a few days. Some practitioners of fasting believe that a juice fast is better than a water-only fast, especially for those who are already nutrient-deficient. Juices have their own cleansing effect, and provide enzymes for detoxification. Juice fasts have been shown to have astounding results, comparable to those of Herbert Shelton's.

A juice fast of three days will cleanse the blood and help the body to eliminate toxins, while a five-day fast will have further-reaching benefits. Fasting on juice for one day a week is also highly recommended. Apple, carrot, grape, beetroot, celery and cabbage are all good to use during a juice fast; avoid orange and tomato juice. For comprehensive details on how to do short juice and other fasts, consult Leon Chaitow's *Thorson's Principles of Fasting* or another of the many books available on the subject.

Colonic irrigation

Colonic irrigation appears to be an effective way of removing substances from the body that may otherwise stay in it until a person's (early) death. Items such as long, black rubbery tubing, a blue marble, fatty lumps, brown stringy objects, rubbery nuggets and gristle have variously been reported as appearing in the post-irrigation debris.[1] At the same time, people have reported health benefits such as shedding mysterious lumps, getting rid of allergies, gaining high energy levels, losing sinus problems, and having clear skin and bright, clear eyes as a result of combining fasting with colonic irrigation.[2]

Hardened mucus builds up in our colons when we eat foods that are hard to digest, such as most of those in the SAD (Standard American Diet), namely cooked meat, white flour, sugar and fats. Around 95 per cent of us have colons clogged with rubbery, black mucus, according to the great pioneer of colon cleansing Dr V. E. Irons. In his *Healthview Newsletter*, Irons has written: 'We have had specimens preserved in alcohol from several inches to a few feet in length, whilst the longest we have had was 27 feet, in one piece. Sometimes it will come out as a pile weighing as much as 11 pounds and continuing to come out for several days to a week . . .'

The subject of colonic irrigation is a hotly debated one, and nutritionists tend to fall between two stools (poor things) as to whether or not it should be done. The populations discussed in this book certainly do not attend irrigation clinics, but then they don't really need to. Herbert Shelton did not use colonic irrigation; but other detoxification clinics believe that it greatly enhances the process of fasting. Some nutritionists object to it on the grounds that washing out your colon strips the mucosal lining and friendly flora.

Its exponents, on the other hand, believe that there is no point in changing to a healthy diet until you have flushed out the system completely; after all, you would not put new engine oil into your car engine without first draining it of the old, filthy stuff. In the end, you will have to make your own decision, based on talking to others, reading about the subject, and perhaps trying it out once and seeing how you feel.

Sweat it out

In her book *Poisoning Our Children*, author Nancy Sokol Green writes of her extraordinary experience of sweating out toxins: 'On the fourteenth day of detox, I started experiencing allergic symptoms, such as eyelid swelling, while I was in the sauna! . . . I was actually beginning to reek of the pesticides that had been sprayed in my home . . . Several of the patients at the clinic who were sensitive to pesticides had to stay away from me as I triggered adverse reactions in them.'[3]

As Green found, we can sweat out copious quantities of waste through our skin, which is why this wonderful organ of detoxification is sometimes called the 'third kidney'. In her book

Digestive Wellness, Elizabeth Lipski recommends low-temperature saunas and steam baths as the most effective methods of sweating out deeply embedded toxins such as pesticides and pharmaceutical drugs from our fatty cells. Another benefit of saunas is that cancer cells dislike heat and die at around 104 degrees Fahrenheit, whereas healthy cells survive.

For detoxification, a sauna needs to be at a fairly low temperature of between 110 and 120 degrees Fahrenheit – you should to be able to stay in for about forty-five minutes, sweating slowly and steadily, without getting too hot. You should do this three to five times weekly so as to keep the momentum going.

Exercise will also help to sweat out toxins. Long-lived populations do not use saunas, but they live in warm climates and take a lot of exercise, so they get plenty of opportunity to sweat out any toxins they may have in their bodies.

Drink water

We may be able to go without food for forty days or more, but without water it would all be over in three to five days. Whether or not you are fasting, it is absolutely essential that you drink plenty of water. It transports nutrients around the body and flushes wastes out. Without it we would drown in a stagnant pool of our own metabolic waste. Water is essential for helping the liver with its taxing job of detoxification, and it is also needed for digestion, circulation, absorption and excretion. Headaches often result from lack of water, as this allows toxins to build up in the system. Water will also keep your skin hydrated and looking younger. You should drink at least eight to ten glasses of water daily, and more when taking exercise, sweating or detoxifying.

Exercise regularly

As well as helping you to sweat out toxins (*see above*), exercise stimulates the lymph function and circulation, thus getting the waste drainage system in your body working properly. No detoxification programme would be complete without it. See Chapter 19 for more about why regular exercise is essential for health and longevity.

IN SUMMARY

Detoxification

- Many great physicians have claimed that *all* illness is caused by toxicity.

- We store toxins in our tissues.

- Our bodies have powerful inbuilt natural healing mechanisms, and fasting is an effective way to allow these mechanisms to work.

- Long-term water fasts have been found to be effective even for serious illness.

- Short juice or water fasts or long-term juice fasts are good options.

- Take low-level saunas to sweat out toxins.

- Drink plenty of water.

- Exercise regularly to boost circulation and lymph drainage.

15

Be immune to ageing

•

W E ALL KNOW PEOPLE who seem to get ill all the time, catching a new cold as soon as the last one has finished, while others 'miraculously' avoid getting anything. Getting ill is not so much to do with whether or not there is disease around (there always is), but with whether or not you can keep it out with a strong immune system.

A weak immune system is also a sign of ageing. By the age of fifty, our immune systems are operating at only a fraction of their efficiency in, say, our twenties, and we start to be much more susceptible to cancer and other illnesses. By taking care of your immune system you can slow your rate of ageing and ward off illness.

Long-lived populations do all the right things in this respect. They eat nutrient-rich, balanced diets, and avoid toxins from junk food and pollution. They get plenty of exercise, and they avoid stress. There *are* many elements of their lifestyles that you can incorporate into your own with a bit of effort. All of the 'secrets' you have read about so far will help you to have a strong immune system, and here I provide you with more tips for boosting your immunity.

The immune system – your personal army

We are all surrounded by pathogens, or disease-causing agents, which would like to get inside us and take over. Your body is like a very desirable fortress on the top of a hill with beautiful views and fertile grounds, and every day the neighbouring armies try to come up the hill and get inside. Whether or not they do depends mainly on the strength of your defences, otherwise known as the immune system.

If your body is a fortress, your skin is its walls and battlements. Pathogens can get in through your mouth and other orifices, however, so your mucus, stomach acid, saliva and vaginal juices act as a kind of moat containing acids and antibodies which invaders have to cross or swim through at their peril. If they manage to get past this hurdle, pathogens will encounter the next wave of defence, your white blood cells. The most ferocious of these are called natural killer cells or NK cells.

NK cells are like millions of James Bonds inside the body, destroying indiscriminately any foreign bodies they chance to come across, especially tumour cells and cells that have been invaded by viruses. There are also phagocytes, which patrol the bloodstream and tissues, engulfing invaders and swallowing them whole; and antibodies are proteins that go to the bloodstream and try to stop viruses from entering body cells.

Like all successful military outfits, the immune system relies on good communication among its staff so that it can work together efficiently. The immune system's army needs equipment to fight with and fuel to keep white blood cells going. We also need to keep our immune systems in top condition so as to defeat the invaders that are continually trying to find ways to outwit them. The human immuno-deficiency virus (HIV), for example, mutates continually, like a secret agent who changes his or her passport and identity every month, making it difficult to fight off. In order to win the battles continually going on inside us, we need to get the right nutrients and avoid stressors on the immune system.

Avoiding illness

According to Patrick Bouic, coauthor of *The Immune System Cure*, 'poor diet is believed to be the main cause of the mal-functioning immune system that accounts for 40 to 70 per cent of all cancers'.[1] Since tumour cells do not carry antigens, or marker tags, identifying them as foreigners, it is important that natural killer cells are in good shape so that they can recognise cancerous cells and destroy them. Some cancers are triggered by viruses such as *Helicobacter pylori* in the stomach and the papilloma virus (herpes) in the cervix. A good diet will build a healthy immune system to help protect you against these types of cancer.

When the immune system reacts against something seemingly harmless like animal dander, pollen or shellfish, the result is an allergic response. One reason why allergic responses such as asthma are on the increase may be that the immune systems of the population as a whole are in a state of decline. Many experts believe that allergic people typically have an imbalance in a certain type of immune cell called T-cells.

Autoimmune diseases such as lupus and rheumatoid arthritis occur when the immune system becomes confused and turns against our own body cells. Certain pathogens confuse the immune system like this by making themselves look like 'self' cells; again, weaker immune systems are more susceptible.

Autoimmune diseases tend to occur after a bout of stress or illness, when the immune system has taken a knock. Orthodox treatment involves suppressing the immune system, which obviously carries major drawbacks; a more sensible solution would be to strengthen the immune system through the good diet and lifestyle practices discussed below.

Five steps to a rejuvenated immune system

We have poor immune systems because they are underfed and overworked. Poor diet, too many toxins, stress and a sedentary lifestyle – in other words, many of the ingredients that go into making up twenty-first-century life – conspire together to wear out our immune system's defences. In order to rejuvenate your immune system, follow the five steps below.

1. EAT IMMUNE-SYSTEM-BOOSTING FOODS

- *Fruit and vegetables* provide antioxidants that support the immune system by neutralising free radicals (see Chapter 7). They also provide vitamins and minerals, such as vitamin C and zinc, which enhance immune system function.

- *Fibre* from fruits, vegetables and whole grains supports the immune system by removing toxins from the body.

- *Whole grains* also provide B vitamins, zinc and selenium, which are all essential for a healthy immune system.

- *Protein* is used to make immune cells, so make sure you eat vegetable protein in the form of tofu, nuts, lentils, quinoa and/or beans. Animal protein is high in saturated fats, which promote tumour growth and clog up the lymphatic (drainage) system, so keep intake to a minimum.

● *Essential fatty acids* from fish and nuts and seeds decrease the inflammation caused by autoimmune disease and enhance the immune system by stimulating T-cells and making tumour necrosis factor. Fish and nuts also provide zinc and the powerful antioxidant selenium.

● *Green tea* has antioxidant, antibiotic and antiviral properties.

● *Water* is needed to flush out toxins and transport nutrients around the body.

● *Shiitake and maitake mushrooms* contain substances called beta-glucan polysaccharides, which boost the immune system deeply and in the long term.

● *Yoghurt* contains friendly flora such as *Lactobacillus bulgaricus*, *bifidobacterium*, and *Lactobacillus acidophilus*, which make their own antibacterial and anti-fungal substances in the gut.

● *Garlic* is a wonderful natural antibiotic; swallowing a clove of raw garlic is an excellent way to get rid of pathogens in the digestive tract. It is also antioxidant, anti-viral and anti-inflammatory; it stimulates the production of natural killer cells, and it is anti-mutagenic.

In addition, you should take a supplement that includes zinc, selenium, the B vitamins, and vitamins A, C and E (see Chapter 18 for more on supplements).

2. AVOID IMMUNE SYSTEM STRESSORS

- *Toxins* from cigarette smoke, junk foods, alcohol and pollution stress out the immune system by giving it extra work to do.

- *Excess sugar* in the blood due to eating sugary foods or refined carbohydrates causes phagocytes to become fat and sluggish.[2] Sugar also raises levels of the 'fight-or-flight' hormones, adrenalin and cortisone, which causes the immune system to lay down tools during the imagined 'emergency' – even a single teaspoon of sugar can suppress the immune system for six hours.

- *Excess insulin* from refined carbohydrates or overeating raises insulin levels, which depresses the immune system.

- *Saturated fats and hydrogenated fats* clog up the lymphatic vessels, effectively crippling your drainage system, and inhibiting the mobility of white blood cells.

- *Alcohol* robs the body of the B vitamins and zinc that are needed for immune-system function; research reveals that red wine drunk in moderation, however, does not seem to have the same effect.

3. THINK YOUR WAY TO BETTER IMMUNITY

Our state of mind has immense power to affect our immune-system function, because our immune systems are hardwired into our nervous systems, which regulate emotions. People are more susceptible to illness, infection, or even death after a stressful life event. Loss of a spouse, considered by psychologists to be the most stressful life event possible, has been found to cause depression and a decline in immune-system function, with many people exhibiting the same symptoms as the dead spouse had during their last illness. Stress also causes the release of certain hormones, such as adrenalin, which suppress the immune-system function.

You can think your way into a state of well-being, even if there are some stressful factors in your real life (and let's face it, when are there not?). Positive thinking and assertiveness are linked with an increase in natural killer cell strength. In a 1996 study, Dr Lee Berk and Dr Stanley Tan gave ten healthy, fasting male volunteers a funny one-hour video to watch, taking blood samples both before and afterwards. They found that even into the next day, there was increased activity in the volunteers' immune systems. Treat yourself to a spot of retail therapy or anything else that you think will help you to think positively; don't feel guilty about it – you are doing it for your immune system.

4. GET PLENTY OF SLEEP

You may have noticed that you are much more susceptible to illness when you are run down. Sleep deprivation lowers natural killer cell activity, while immune-system function is improved with good-quality sleep, during which potent immune-system-enhancing compounds are released.

If you are unable to get a good eight hours' sleep at night, you could try meditating to make up some of the deficit. As well as being very relaxing, meditation has been found to enhance T-cell activity.[3] Alternatively, try lying on the bed and listening to some relaxing music. Certain rhythmic patterns and harmonies have been found in experiments to increase levels of the 'youth hormone' DHEA, reduce the stress hormone cortisol and raise the levels of certain anti-bodies.[4]

5. EXERCISE REGULARLY

No immune-system-enhancing diet and lifestyle programme would be complete without moderate daily exercise. Exercise raises natural killer cell activity and keeps the muscles pushing your lymph around the lymphatic vessels. Particularly good forms of immune-system-boosting exercise are brisk walking, yoga, and t'ai chi; the latter has been found to increase white blood cell production by up to 40 per cent.

Too much exercise can be detrimental to the immune system, however – it is a well-documented fact that serious athletes such as marathon runners are often immune-system-suppressed and frequently fall prey to colds and infections. Too much exercise can damage tissues, resulting in inflammation, and it also raises free radical production. Athletes have been found to have reduced NK cell activity and lowered levels of DHEA.[5]

IN SUMMARY

Your immune system

- A strong immune system is a sign of a youthful body.

- Eat a balanced, nutrient-rich diet that includes plenty of fruits, vegetables, whole grains and essential fats.

- Take an antioxidant supplement and/or multi-nutrient supplement.

- Avoid or restrict stressors of the immune system such as toxins, sugar, caffeine, saturated fats and alcohol.

- Try to reduce stress and be a positive thinker.

- Get plenty of sleep and relaxation.

- Take regular exercise such as a brisk twenty-minute daily walk or some form of exercise class.

16

Eat food for thought

•

... here he was, with his head bulging at the back and on his face that look of quiet intelligence which comes from eating lots of fish.

P.G. WODEHOUSE, British humorous novelist, 1881–1975,
Bertie Wooster in *Stiff Upper Lip, Jeeves*

OUR BRAINS ARE MADE OF FOOD, and what we eat or drink can affect how we think, feel and behave. If you have ever felt sugar highs and lows, or watched people coming out of a pub at closing time, you will know this to be so. Serene dispositions and impressive mental acuity, even into very old age, have often been noted in the long-lived people discussed in Part I. The authors of the Okinawa study, for example, found that most Okinawans had 'remarkable mental clarity' even past the age of a hundred, while visitors to Hunza have particularly stressed the happy dispositions of Hunzakuts of all ages.

In the West, on the other hand, mental illness is rising to

epidemic proportions. A World Health Organisation conference in 2002 revealed that 450 million people suffer from mental problems such as depression, schizophrenia or dementia, which makes mental and neurological illnesses among the top causes of ill health in the West.

Of course, not all mental health is directly related to nutrition. However, there is an established link between diet and mental health. According to the Okinawa study authors, the low rates of dementia among Okinawans are thought to be mainly due to dietary habits.[1] Likewise Robert McCarrison's experiments with rats fed a Hunza-type diet showed how dramatically diet can affect mood and behaviour (*see page 74*). In a recent trial at a young offenders' institution in Britain, it was found that supplementing with vitamins, minerals and essential fatty acids resulted in a huge drop in serious offences of 40 per cent.

Your brain cells do not always die off permanently with age, as was once thought.[2] This means that you have some control over the rate at which your brain ages. The way to keep your brain young is to give it the right fuel. As you will see, keeping your brain youthful means doing most of the same things you have to do to keep the rest of you young and healthy, which isn't really surprising since the brain is an integral part of the body.

Fish for brains

If anyone ever calls you a fathead, you can thank them for the compliment. Around 60 per cent of our brains are made of fats, especially the omega 3 essential fatty acid derivative DHA (docosahexaenoic acid), otherwise known as the 'brain fat'. It has even been suggested that it was our ancestors' fishy diet that was responsible for transforming the primate-sized brains we had five or six million years ago into the large, intelligent brains we house inside our craniums now, which are capable of composing symphonies and making nuclear bombs.

Omega 3 fats are needed for the production of neurotransmitters, brain chemicals that regulate states such as mood and libido. Two other parts of the body that rely on DHA for proper functioning are the retina of the eye and the central nervous system, which is our brain and spinal cord. In other words, DHA is essential for proper thinking, feeling, seeing and motor coordination. The best source of DHA is oily fish such as salmon, mackerel, tuna and sardines. No wonder fish is such an important component of the diets studied in this book.

The last trimester and the first twelve months of life are the most important for our brain development, with our brains tripling in size by our first birthday, so it is important that we get a good intake of DHA during that time. Happily, nature has organised it so that this is precisely what happens, by making sure that breast-feeding infants milk their mothers of all the DHA they can get via the breast.

Breast-fed babies score on average 3 to 5 points higher on the IQ scale than formula-fed babies, which is a great deal when you consider that 5 IQ points can make the difference between being 'educationally subnormal' and 'normal'. It is for this reason that many brands of formula milk now contain added DHA, and these formulas have been found to improve the cognitive ability of infants.[3]

Because both a foetus and a baby take its mother's supply of DHA, pregnant and lactating women who do not get enough DHA in their diets often become deficient. It is now thought that this may cause post-natal depression. Pregnant and lactating women should eat oily fish at least twice a week or supplement with 200–400 mg daily of DHA for this reason. DHA is available in vegan form, which may be best for pregnant women since fish liver oil contains high levels of vitamin A and this can be toxic to a foetus. Fish oil should also not be fed directly to infants as it has been shown in some studies to impair mental development, for reasons that are not yet clear.

DHA and cognitive development

Getting enough DHA is also important for older children. Children who were breast-fed as infants have a lower incidence of problems such as dyslexia and dyspraxia, while studies have shown that children with dyspraxia improve noticeably when given DHA supplements.[4]

Around one in twenty children in the UK have attention deficit hyperactivity disorder (ADHD), a condition that makes the lives of both parents and teachers a misery. Children performing such antics as leaping over banisters to try and fly, sleeping only two hours a night or attempting to stab their siblings are regularly reported in the press.

ADHD is characterised by low levels of the neurotransmitter dopamine, which relies on DHA for production. An Oxford University study found that children with ADHD had essential fatty acid deficiency, and showed the rough dry skin and dry hair which are clinical signs of deficiency. After being given fish oil supplements for three months, DHA levels in the children's brains recovered, and the researchers found 'stark' differences in markers such as ability to pay attention, relaxation and emotional volatility.

DHA and depression

If you suffer from chronic depression without knowing why, you may benefit from DHA supplementation. When Andrew

Stoll and colleagues gave fish oil to patients with manic depression, they saw 'dramatic differences' in their subjects; improvements were so striking the study was ended several months early.[5] One reason for this may be that DHA raises levels of serotonin, the anti-depressive neurotransmitter.[6]

In the well-known Framingham Study, which looked at the link between low cholesterol levels and heart disease, researchers were dismayed to find that those with a low dietary intake of cholesterol were more likely to be depressed or to commit suicide that those with a higher intake. This is why those who are on a low-fat diet should make sure that they do not exclude essential fatty acids.

The importance of antioxidants

If you eat a lot of fish or take DHA supplements, your DHA-rich brain cells will be especially vulnerable to free radical damage, so it is absolutely essential that you get enough of the fat-soluble antioxidants vitamins E and A, which get into cell membranes and protect them from damage.[7]

You also need to get plenty of antioxidants in order to prevent free radical damage to the arteries leading to your brain, so that your brain can get all the nutrients it needs. Vitamins A, C and E are particularly important (see Chapter 7 on antioxidants). The Okinawans get much of their vitamin E from sweet potatoes, while the Symiots and Campodimelani get theirs from olive oil.

A helping of salmon or mackerel with a salad of avocado, carrots, baby spinach leaves, and an olive oil and garlic dressing is a good brain meal containing both DHA and vitamins E and A. It is also a good idea to take a vitamin E supplement as it is hard to get enough vitamin E from food. Also drink green tea; this contains the fat-soluble antioxidant epigallocatechin-gallate, which is thought to be even more effective than vitamin E at protecting brain cells. The antioxidants proantho-cyanidins, found in red wine and red berries, also protect brain cells from free radical damage.

How B vitamins help

Do you find that you sometimes forget what you came into the room for or where you parked your car, or feel confused, anxious or depressed? It could be due to a simple lack of B vitamins. Several studies have found that up to a third of those who appear to have mild dementia are actually suffering from vitamin B12 deficiency and can make a full recovery with B12 supplements, the reason being that B12 is needed to make the neurotransmitters involved in memory recall.[8] Vitamin B12 deficiency is also thought to be linked to multiple sclerosis, as the vitamin is needed for maintaining the myelin sheath around nerve fibres in the central nervous system.

For good mental health you need to get enough of all the B vitamins together. The B vitamin choline, for example, makes the memory neurotransmitter acetylcholine with the help of vitamin B5, which is itself known as the anti-stress vitamin. Folic acid helps to make the neurotransmitters dopamine and serotonin, and has been found to help schizophrenic and depressed patients.[9]

Good sources of B vitamins are whole grains, fish and meat; if in doubt, take a B complex supplement (the populations discussed earlier get theirs mainly from whole grains and fish). Strict vegans should take extra care to obtain enough vitamin B12; only tiny amounts are needed, but animal products and fish are virtually the only source.

Keeping the digestive system healthy

It is crucial that you keep your gut happy so that it can service the nutrient-guzzling organ at the top properly. The brain runs on large amounts of glucose, which the gut must provide by breaking down carbohydrates efficiently, and it also needs other nutrients, which must be extracted from food in the stomach and intestine. The gut must also be able to detoxify the body, so that toxins do not end up in the circulation and thence in the brain, where they damage brain cells and cause 'brain fog' or worse.

It is estimated that up to 93 per cent of migraines are caused by sensitivities and allergies to foods such as dairy products, wheat, citrus fruits, shellfish, eggs and tomatoes, possibly because allergic reactions cause inflammation in the blood vessels around the brain. Autism has also been linked with food sensitivities – perhaps because culprits such as wheat and dairy products produce proteins called peptides that pass through a permeable gut and act like opiates on the brain. Hyperactivity in children may also be caused by food sensitivites.[10] People with ADHD have often been found to have problems with their guts such as food allergies and excess gut permeability, or leaky gut syndrome.

How a raw food diet may help

When Leslie and Susannah Kenton, authors of *Raw Energy: Eat Your Way to Radiant Health*, changed to a mainly raw diet they found that they could think more clearly, had greater confidence and stopped suffering from bouts of depression.[11] One reason for this may be the effects a detoxifying diet has on our brains – no more toxins means no more poisonous thoughts.

A high-raw food diet also helps to balance blood sugar levels, which means no more mood swings. A dietary day consisting of going to the office, drinking coffee, coming home, losing your temper, then eating three pastries will have the opposite effect. A diet high in the refined carbohydrates that cause blood sugar swings has also been found to dramatically lower IQ scores.[12] Even worse, it produces advanced glycosylation end-products (AGEs) in the brain – these are found at raised levels in Alzheimer's patients.[13]

Why you should avoid meat

A high-meat diet is linked to brain disease such as Parkinson's and Alzheimer's. When the blood vessels are clogged due to you eating saturated fats, the brain gets deprived of nutrients and is more susceptible to free radical damage and other problems. In a recent study at Newcastle University it was found that 80 per cent of Alzheimer's patients had heart disease; the researchers suggested that narrowed blood vessels had starved subjects' brains of nutrients. Blocked blood vessels can also cause strokes to the brain. The people described in Part I have youthful blood vessels unclogged by saturated fats; they have both good brain health and good heart health as a result.

Keeping the brain active

If you hate jogging, take heart from the fact that sitting comfortably on a sofa while exercising the mind can keep you young and make you more intelligent. Doing crosswords has been found to improve the immune system by boosting antibody production, which means fending off degenerative disease. Studies also show that our brains can be exercised just like our other muscles and can continue to grow and perform throughout our lives. A University College London survey, for example, found that in London's black taxi drivers, the part of the brain where maps and street names are stored in the memory is larger compared with the same part of the brain in other people (although the rest of their brains are no bigger than anyone else's).[14]

Doing an activity you enjoy, such as going on a weekend trip or attending a concert, creates endorphins. This boosts circulation to the brain, so that it gets more oxygen and nutrients. Aerobic exercise has the same effect, and is thought to be able to raise IQ by several points. As an experiment, try deep breathing and see if you can feel an increase in your mental acuity: breathe in for eight counts, hold your breath for twelve, exhale for ten, and repeat ten times, stopping if you feel dizzy. This will have the additional benefit of relieving stress, which causes the release of brain-ageing cortisol.

IN SUMMARY

Keeping your brain young

- Your brain is a growing, active organ that requires sustenance and exercise, just like the rest of your body. By giving it what it needs, you can keep it young and healthy even into old age.

- Eat oily fish regularly or take DHA supplements to provide your brain with the building blocks it needs.

- Ensure a good antioxidant intake so as to protect the vulnerable fatty acids in your brain from free radical damage.

- Take a B vitamin complex and eat plenty of vitamin B-rich foods to protect against neurological disease.

- Look after your gut so that it can provide the brain with the nutrients it needs.

- Avoid a high-glycaemic diet of refined carbohydrates and sugary products to prevent mood swings and AGEs.

- Restrict intake of saturated fats such as meat and dairy products to keep the blood vessels to the brain clear.

- Exercise your brain to keep it agile, and do activities you enjoy.

- Take regular aerobic exercise for increased circulation to the brain.

chapter

17

Eat organic and avoid Frankenfoods

•

If we don't change the direction in which we are going,
we will end up where we are headed.

RED SKELTON, US artist and writer

THE LONG-LIVED PEOPLE described in Part I are organic
farmers par excellence. They do not use pesticides, artificial fertilisers, or genetically modified (GM) crops. Yet
their yields are abundant, their crops are healthy, their soil is
rich and they do not have problems with insect 'pests' because
these are eaten by other insects and birds. The Hunzakuts in
particular are famous for their skilful manure-making and
other farming methods, and their health has been attributed by
some researchers to the high quality of their soil. When soil is
healthy and rich in minerals, the plants that grow on it are
also healthy and rich in minerals, as are the humans who then
eat those plants.

Why farm organic?

Using artificial fertilisers and pesticides has been very seductive to commercial farmers, as they increase the quantity of crops in the short term. In the long term, however, they cause the soil and crops to become dependent upon them, much as a person given medicine may become dependent on it and need more and more of it while their health continues to decline. Artificial fertilisers drain the soil of valuable minerals such as calcium and magnesium, so that the food that is grown on it cannot provide us with them. They also leach nitrates into drinking water, and these are converted into carcinogens in our bodies.

It is true that when pesticides are first introduced into a farming environment, insects literally drop from the crops and yields initially increase as a result. Over time, however, while the weaker species of insect die out, the hardier ones adapt and evolve pesticide-resistant strains, which are stronger and more damaging to the crops than the original strains. According to John Robbins, author of *Diet For a New America,* the percentage of US crops lost to insects doubled between 1950 and 1974, mostly because pesticides disturbed the ecological balance.[1]

A typical lettuce has been sprayed with pesticides twelve times by the time it reaches the supermarket shelf.[2] When you eat fruits and vegetables that have been sprayed, your body is able (by using up much of its precious energy) to detoxify to a certain extent, but many toxins accumulate in your body tissues. Eating meat is the worst thing you can do, because chemicals from sprayed grains concentrate in the flesh of animal tissue. Women's breast milk tends to have concentrated levels of pesticides, although vegetarian mothers have far lower levels than ones who eat meat.[3] Pesticide use has been suggested as one cause of the increased rates of child cancer in the last fifty years and the incidence of illnesses such as mild cognitive disorder in gardeners and farmers.[4]

Organic farming methods

Organic farmers spread manure and compost over the soil, which ensures that the nutrients that are taken out of it are put back in. Crop rotation prevents crops from draining the soil of minerals needed to grow those crops. Pests are kept away with natural, harmless methods – for example, fruit orchards are kept free of whitefly by introducing beetles that do not eat the fruits and only eat the flies, while hedgerows encourage the presence of birds and insects, which feed on pests. Healthy crops grown on rich soil are also more able to resist disease.

The soil used in organic farming is bountiful and fertile in the long term. Organically grown food is better for health and has more flavour than food produced in an intensive way because it contains more nutrients, which have been taken up from the rich soil. The soil in Bama, for example, has been found to be high in manganese and zinc, and hair-analysis tests have shown that these same minerals are at the right levels for optimum heart health in the Bama people. According to The Soil Association in the UK, 'research comparing the nutrient contents of organic and non-organic fruit and vegetables reveals a strong trend towards higher levels in organic produce'.

Organic produce still has a way to go. It is more expensive than non-organic produce and is not as widely accessible as it could be. The amount of money the UK government has put into promoting organic farming is minuscule compared with how much it has invested in more modern, hi-tech farming methods. Yet organic farming is often best for the consumer, the farmer and the environment, especially in the long term. By buying organic when you can, and encouraging your local supermarket to promote organic foods, you will help improve your own health and that of the planet.

The 'Frankenfoods'

Genetic modification, in which scientists take genes from one organism and put them into another, is a very complicated process with unknown effects. 'We're right at the very beginning of this incredible set of scientific advances,' the chief technology officer for Monsanto, Robb Fraley, recently proclaimed.[5] They certainly are. Genetic modification science is still in its infancy, and much more experimentation needs to be done before it is fully understood – if it *can* ever be fully understood. It is us and the natural environment, which took millions of years to evolve in a very specific way, that will be the guinea pigs in this vast, unpredictable experiment. At least we can wash pesticides off under the tap; we cannot do this with genes.

Most studies on GM foods have been undertaken by the companies that want to profit from developing them, and have been kept from the public.[6] However, the studies that are available show worrying findings.

When Dr Arpad Pusztai of the Rowett Research Institute in Aberdeen fed rats with potatoes that had been genetically modified to contain lectin, he found that one group of rats showed suppressed immune systems, slight growth retardation and changes in internal organ weights. Adding lectin to ordinary potatoes and feeding them to rats produced no ill-effects, indicating that it was the process of genetic modification itself, rather than the lectin, that did the damage. In another study by GM giant Aventis, chickens fed with GM maize were twice as likely to die as those fed non-GM maize.[7]

Why grow GM crops?

What are GM crops for anyway? The people discussed earlier certainly have no use for them. Neither do the commercial Asian farmers who have become disillusioned with them.[8] GM crops have nothing to do with feeding the world, and everything to do with profit. The GM companies themselves admit this: Steve Smith of GM giant Novartis recently said, 'If anyone tells you GM is going to feed the world, tell him that it is not. To feed the world takes political and financial will, it's not about production and distribution. It may produce more for less and create more food but it won't feed the world.'

GM companies like to advertise the fact that they are developing crops with added vitamins to combat malnutrition, yet the reality is that most GM crop development in countries such as the UK, Australia and South Africa is focused on commodity crops such as oilseed rape, cotton, soya and maize, destined for the lucrative mass market.

Most of the GM crops currently being developed in the UK are weedkiller tolerant, which means that heavy doses of chemicals can be used to spray the fields they are in, killing the weeds but not the crops. There is widespread concern that the use of weedkiller-tolerant GM crops will encourage the evolution of 'superweeds' – triffid-like weeds that can adapt to survive the sprays and cause environmental havoc such as the eradication of native bird species.[9]

Research shows that GM crops can interbreed with wild plants and contaminate them with their genes.[10] GM crops are thought to be able to contaminate non-GM crops growing up to nine kilometres away. This means that if GM farms are set up near to organic farms, the organic farms will go out of business. GM crops also have a nasty habit of entering the food chain in unpredictable ways. In a disastrous case in the US, StarLink, a variety of GM corn intended purely for animal feed due to concern that it might cause allergic reactions, somehow found its way into taco shells on supermarket shelves.

As many as 77 per cent of people in the UK do not want GM crops to be grown, according to a 1998 MORI poll. In November 2002 the British Medical Association issued a statement saying 'There has not yet been a robust and thorough search into the potentially harmful effects of GM foodstuffs on human health. On the basis of the precautionary principle, farm-scale trials should not be allowed to continue.' Yet commercial growing has already begun in the UK, and at the time of writing there are 178 farm trials of GM crops being carried out; the biotech companies envisage a future in which the UK is 'carpeted' in GM crops.[11]

What you can do

If you want to avoid the potential health risks of having pesticides in your body, buy organic food when you can, or grow your own if you have spare time and space. Limit the amount of meat and dairy products you eat, especially non-organic types, as these contain the most concentrated levels of pesticides and antibiotics. Make sure you scrub fruits and vegetables well under the tap before eating them. Supermarkets listen to their consumers – they need to – so encourage your local supermarkets and greengrocers to stock organic produce, and non-organic produce treated only with pesticides that do not leave residues.

To avoid eating GM produce, check the labels on foods carefully. Soya, corn products and foods containing oilseed rape are the most likely foods to contain GM produce – processed foods in particular are likely to contain them. If you want to support the campaign for a five-year freeze on GM crops, write to your local MP and consult an environmental campaign group for details (*see* Resources, *page 285* for contacts).

IN SUMMARY

Organic versus non-organic foods

- Pesticides and artificial fertilisers damage the health of soil and crops – and by extension, you.

- Organic produce has measurably higher levels of vitamins and minerals than non-organic produce.

- The long-term effects of GM crops have not been tested; the independent tests that have been taken indicate risks to health.

- Buy organic when you can and avoid eating produce contaminated with pesticides or GM crops; wash any sprayed produce thoroughly.

Supplement your diet

•

THE LONG-LIVED POPULATIONS discussed in Part I do not need to take vitamin and mineral supplements because their soil is rich and fertile, and full of nutrients. By contrast, the soil that supports our crops (and animals) has been drained of nutrients by intensive farming methods, as we've just seen in the previous chapter.

The supplements controversy

In 2002 the UK press reported that, according to the results of a major Oxford University study, supplements are a waste of money. In the study, it was claimed that 20,000 people who were given supplements of vitamin E, vitamin C and beta-carotene for five years did not show any improvement in health. Yet these vitamins have also been found by the same university to cut crime among juvenile offenders. In another study by the US National Institute of Aging, it was found that among 10,000 elderly people, taking vitamins C and E halved the risk of dying from any cause.

What is going on? At the same time that the Oxford University study came out, the pharmaceuticals giants were (and still are) lobbying for high licensing costs for smaller supplement manufacturers, which would force most of them to go under. Just before the Oxford University study, the UK government announced that supplements are unnecessary 'as part of a balanced diet'. But junk food is also unnecessary as part of a balanced diet, yet the government doesn't seem to be forcing hot-dog stands out business.

Why we may need supplements

My view is that – contrary to the government's advice – many of us may need supplements. Our food can only be as good as the soil it is grown in and, thanks to modern farming methods, it is no longer much good at all. An orange you buy in the supermarket today can contain as little as zero vitamin C, while the magnesium levels in carrots have dropped by 75 per cent since 1940. You need a minimum of 400 grams of vitamin C daily to ward off colds and more serious illnesses such as cancer and heart disease, and if you have low magnesium levels you are at risk of suffering from heart irregularities.

Most of us are not getting the vitamins and minerals, or micronutrients, we need. There are at least seventeen minerals and thirteen vitamins that are essential for health and that we need to obtain from our food. In 1988, the US Surgeon-General concluded in his *Report on Health and Nutrition* that around 75 per cent of deaths in the United States involved nutritional deficiencies. Unless you get your vegetables from mineral-rich soil that has been carefully fertilised with natural composts and manures for many years, as the people discussed in Part I do, you almost certainly need to take vitamin and mineral supplements for optimum health.

Anti-ageing supplements

Below is an outline of some of the main anti-ageing vitamins and minerals available in supplement form. If you take a good multivitamin and mineral supplement you can get a good range of essential vitamins and minerals, including these, without having to think about which one is supposed to do what. Remember that supplements are just that – they are supposed to supplement a balanced diet, not replace it. A cheeseburger, chips and a milk shake followed by a handful of pills will not lead to optimum health.

If you have ever looked at the Recommended Daily Allowance (RDA) amounts on the side of a jar of vitamins, you will notice that the suggested dosages given here are *much* higher. RDA levels are set by government scientists and are based on how much of a given nutrient is needed to prevent serious deficiency diseases such as scurvy and beri-beri, rather than on how much is needed for optimum health.

Vitamin C

Vitamin C is a potent immune-system-boosting antioxidant that is absolutely essential for our good health in many ways. The champion of vitamin C, Nobel prizewinner Dr Linus Pauling, claimed that we could add twelve to eighteen years to our lives if we took 3 to 12 grams of vitamin C daily; he himself claimed to have lived an extra twenty years because of the large doses of vitamin C he took.

Vitamin C quenches carcinogenic free radicals and protects DNA from being damaged. According to Gladys Block, cancer epidemiologist at the University of California, Berkeley, people who eat the highest amounts of vitamin C are half as likely to get cancer as people who are deficient in the vitamin.[1] Vitamin C also builds collagen and protects arteries from damage. A study published in the *British Medical Journal* showed that men who had low levels of vitamin C were three and a half times more likely to have a heart attack than those who did not.[2]

Suggested optimal dose 1,000–3,000 mg (1–3 g) is recommended; 400 mg at the very minimum. Use magnesium ascorbate for best absorption, and spread the dose throughout the day.

Caution No known toxicity, although very high doses can cause diarrhoea. If taking the contraceptive pill, 10 g daily may render it ineffective. Vitamin C aids absorption of iron so if you have a disorder involving inability to handle iron (such as hemochromatosis) consult a doctor.

Food sources Red peppers, berries, citrus fruits and cruciferous vegetables, eaten raw.

Vitamin A/beta-carotene

Once known as the 'anti-infective vitamin', vitamin A and its precursor, beta-carotene, is a major factor in immune-system health. It is a powerful, fat-soluble antioxidant that protects cell membranes and mucus membranes such as those lining the lungs and the digestive tract.

Over a hundred studies have shown that people with high levels of vitamin A are about half as likely as those with low levels to develop various cancers, especially lung cancer.[3] Beta-carotene prevents LDL cholesterol from being oxidised; diets high in beta-carotene have been found to lower the risk of heart attack by up to a half.[4]

Suggested optimal dose 5,000–50,000 iu of beta-carotene or 7,500–20,000 iu vitamin A. For best absorption, beta-carotene and vitamin A should be taken with beneficial fats such as those found in oily fish or olive oil.

Caution Vitamin A can be toxic in very high doses (over 50,000 iu daily). Do not take more than 2,000 iu of vitamin A in pregnancy as it can be toxic to the foetus, although it does need some vitamin A for proper development. You can take much higher levels of beta-carotene as the body will only convert the amount it needs. Beta-carotene is non-toxic although very high levels can cause a slight yellowing of the skin, which is temporary and is thought to be completely harmless.

Food sources Dark green, orange and red fruits and vegetables; cod liver oil, liver.

Vitamin E

Vitamin E has been dubbed the 'fountain of youth' for its heart-protective properties. This powerful fat-soluble anti-oxidant boosts the immune system and protects against heart disease and cancer; high blood levels are associated with health and longevity.[5] Studies show that low blood levels of vitamin E make people 50 per cent more susceptible to all kinds of cancer.[6] Vitamin E also protects the heart by thinning the blood and preventing LDL cholesterol from oxidising; a major study has showed that it can reduce the risk of heart attack by 40 per cent.[7]

Suggested optimal dose 400 iu–800 iu daily; take with vitamin C, which recycles 'spent' vitamin E

Caution If you are taking anticoagulant drugs, consult your doctor. Vitamin E can replace blood-thinning drugs, but this must be done gradually and with care. If you have high blood pressure, consult your doctor before using vitamin E.

Food sources Nuts, fish oil, olive oil, avocados.

Selenium

Selenium rejuvenates the immune system; studies show that the immune systems of older people given selenium behave like those of younger people.[8] It is also a powerful antioxidant; studies have found that cancer death can be reduced by half by taking selenium supplements.[9] High levels of selenium in soil in some places (Norfolk, England and Rumania are two examples) are associated with a reduced risk of cancer, while areas with low selenium levels in the soil have been found to have higher cancer and virus levels.[10]

Selenium protects the heart by boosting the function of the mitochondria, the power-houses of heart cells. In a large-scale study in Finland, it was found that those with the lowest blood levels of selenium were three times more likely to die from heart disease than those with the highest levels.[11]

Suggested optimal dose 100–200 mcg daily.

Caution Selenium can be toxic in high doses of 2,500 mcg daily (liver damage, joint inflammation). Japanese fishermen have around 500 mcg per day without any apparent damage, but keep to 200 mcg daily to be on the safe side.

Food sources Brazil nuts straight from the shell are an excellent source – one or two provide enough selenium for a day. If you buy pre-shelled nuts, you need more, as they come from a different part of Brazil with lower selenium levels. Selenium is also found in garlic, asparagus, seafood and whole grains.

Zinc

Zinc deficiency is very common, especially in elderly people. Look at your fingernails – if you have more than two small white spots in the fingertip part, you are likely to be zinc deficient. Animals with zinc deficiency have been found to have 15 to 20 per cent higher levels of free radicals in their bodies than animals with normal levels.[12] Zinc regulates normal cell death and tells problem cells to 'commit suicide', which prevents them from dividing uncontrollably – an important anti-cancer mechanism. Zinc also has a seemingly miraculous ability to rejuvenate an ageing thymus gland; this gland is responsible for overseeing our all-important immune systems.

Suggested optimal dose 10–30 mg daily. Zinc gluconate is the best-absorbed form.

Caution Do not exceed 50 mg as high doses may interfere with absorption of other nutrients.

Food sources Oysters, meat, poultry, garlic, whole grains, green leafy vegetables, and nuts and seeds.

Coenzyme Q10

Coenzyme Q10 (coQ10) is a powerful anti-ageing antioxidant that is the subject of much exciting new research, particularly with regard to its ability to boost heart health.[13] It is one of the few antioxidants that can get inside the mitochondria, the power houses of our cells which are highly susceptible to free radical damage, particularly in the heart and brain.

Studies show that coQ10 can rejuvenate the immune system in ageing people.[14] It also has antiviral, antibacterial and anti-tumour effects, with some cancer patients showing complete regression.[15] Mice given coQ10 stay younger for longer and are more active in old age, according to studies conducted at UCLA.[16]

Suggested optimal dose 50–100mg or more daily.

Food sources sardines, mackerel, organ meats.

Glutathione

Glutathione is a potent antioxidant that regenerates immune cells and makes them super-efficient. Known as the 'master antioxidant', it is needed by every cell in our bodies. It is abundant in most foods and is produced in our cells, but people who are even moderately deficient are more likely to age prematurely, as free radicals are left unchecked.[17] Levels drop with age: in one study, elderly patients who were given 75 mg daily had a dramatic increase in immune cell activity and they felt healthier and more energetic.[18]

Suggested optimal dose 50–100 mg daily. 500 mg daily of vitamin C boosts glutathione levels.

Food sources Raw fruits and vegetables, especially avocado, watermelon, asparagus, and cruciferous vegetables such as cauliflower and broccoli.

Calcium

This mineral is necessary for bone health, although it cannot work without magnesium and vitamin D. Vitamin D is synthesised in the body from sunlight, and is also found in seafood. Supplementation with vitamin D should not be necessary; however, you do need to ensure adequate magnesium intake.

Suggested optimal dose 500 mg–1,000 mg, taken with magnesium. You may be getting enough from the diet; it is often lack of magnesium which is a problem rather than lack of calcium. Too much calcium also depletes levels of magnesium (*see below*).

Caution Over 2,000 mg can be toxic; too much can cause constipation.

Food sources The best food sources are cruciferous vegetables (such as broccoli), nuts and seeds, as these also contain magnesium. Other sources include kale, yoghurt, alfalfa sprouts, pulses, fish (especially soft bones in canned fish), seaweed, tofu and sardines. Contrary to what many people think, cheese is not the best source of calcium as it lacks magnesium and can cause leaching of calcium from the bones (see Chapter 9).

Magnesium

Magnesium protects the mitochondria in our cells from free radical damage, and this is thought to be at the core of the ageing process. According to French researchers, animals that are deficient in magnesium are almost perfect specimens of accelerated ageing.[19]

Magnesium gives us youthful flexibility. It relaxes and dilates the blood vessels and keeps the muscles, including the heart muscle, flexible; people who die suddenly from heart attacks have been found to have low levels of magnesium.[20] It can also work as a mild laxative by relaxing the smooth muscles lining the colon, and it works with calcium to maintain bone health.

Suggested optimal dose 400–800 mg, depending on your calcium intake – you need half as much magnesium as calcium.

Caution Magnesium relaxes the bowel so avoid large doses if you have diarrhoea. Do not take if you have severe kidney problems or heart failure.

Food sources Whole grains, green leafy vegetables, broccoli, nuts and seeds.

Chromium

Dr Gary Evans of Bemidji State University, Minnesota, says: 'I call chromium the geriatric nutrient because everybody starts to really need it past age 35.' Chromium deficiency, which is extremely common, causes premature ageing; rats given chromium have been found to live longer and have more vitality than those that were not given it. The main function of chromium as an anti-ageing agent is in forming Glucose Tolerance Factor (GTF), which is involved in getting blood glucose into cells. In one study of people with adult-onset diabetes, those given 200 mcg of chromium picolinate daily had their blood sugar levels lowered as effectively as with orthodox medication.[21]

Suggested optimal dose 200 mcg daily in chromium picolinate form.

Food sources Nuts, seeds, whole grains.

B vitamins

You need to take the whole complex of B vitamins in order for your body to metabolise nutrients and make immune cells. Especially important are vitamins B6, B12 and folic acid. B vitamin deficiency is linked with various illnesses of ageing including cancer, heart disease, senility and multiple sclerosis. Vitamin B6 protects the heart by metabolising homocysteine, while B12 deficiency symptoms include memory loss, neurological problems and pernicious anaemia. Folic acid deficiency increases the risk of cancer.[22]

Suggested optimal dose A good supplement will give you levels far higher than the RDAs; choose a good brand for sufficient dosages.

Vitamin B6 food sources Seafood, whole grains, nuts, soya, bananas, sweet potatoes, prunes and poultry.

Folic acid food sources Meat, fish, poultry, grains, nuts and seeds, soya, green leafy vegetables, potatoes, legumes, organ meats, mushrooms and cruciferous vegetables.

Vitamin B12 food sources Meat, fish and poultry.

chapter

19

Exercise, exercise, exercise

•

I read the prescription. It ran:
1 lb beefsteak,
with 1 pt bitter beer every six hours.
1 ten-mile walk every morning.
1 bed at 11 sharp every night.
. . . I followed the directions, with the happy result –
speaking for myself – that my life was preserved, and is still
going on.

JEROME K. JEROME, *Three Men in a Boat*

YOU WILL BE HARD PUSHED to find exceptionally long-lived
people who don't take a lot of exercise. Those described
in Part I all lead outdoor lives, farm, get in the day's
catch, do housework and climb up and down the rugged
terrain in which they live. They are also fond of sports – the
Okinawans practise martial arts, for example, while the
Hunzakuts enjoy regular dancing sessions along with their
home-brewed alcohol. Even the super-centenarians in these

places are mobile and able to take part in some physical activity on most days. There is no doubt that exercise is an integral part of any longevity programme.

According to a recent study, inactivity is an even stronger predictor of death risk than high cholesterol levels, high blood pressure, diabetes and heart disease (which could justify eating a slice of chocolate cake occasionally provided that you take regular exercise!).[1] Exercise is so important for good health that it can even negate some of the harmful effects of smoking. According to a 1996 report in the *Journal of the American Medical Association*, smokers who are moderately fit live longer than sedentary nonsmokers. However, it is only once a nutritious diet is combined with regular exercise that the real benefits occur.

Exercise makes you look and feel better and benefits every part of your body. It reduces the risk of cancer and, according to one study, particularly reduces the risk of colon cancer in men and breast cancer in women.[2] It lowers blood pressure, homocysteine levels and LDL cholesterol levels, so reducing the risk of heart disease: according to a Harvard study, men who run for an hour or more each week lower their risk of heart disease by 42 per cent.[3] All of the muscles in your body, including the heart and those lining the colon, need regular exercise in order to function well.

Exercise boosts the circulation so that more nutrients get to your cells, and it improves lymphatic function so that your waste drainage system works properly. Exercise improves the immune system by boosting white blood cell performance and ridding the body of toxins through sweat. For women, exercise can help prevent a difficult pregnancy and labour, and it reduces the risk of osteoporosis.[4] Exercise will also help you lose weight, through boosting the metabolism as well as burning off a few calories.

There are numerous studies that show that regular, aerobic exercise can add several years to your life. On average, those who live to be a hundred walk an hour a day, or get the equivalent amount of exercise.[5] Growth hormone, associated with youthfulness, is stimulated by exercise. Studies show that regular exercise slows the ageing process by lowering blood glucose levels, which prevents ageing cross-linking and insulin damage to blood vessels.

Even if you aren't overweight, a sedentary lifestyle increases your chances of developing glucose intolerance and diabetes; inactive men are almost four times as likely as active men to get diabetes.[6] People who exercise regularly are also less likely to become disabled in later life.[7] It is never too late to start taking regular exercise; one study by W. J. Evans showed that even people aged ninety-six can increase their strength and muscle size by beginning an exercise programme.

Exercise is good for mental health and happiness. Studies show that exercise improves mood, reduces anxiety and depression, and gets rid of stress.[8] Exercise can even raise your IQ; in one study, older adults who walked for forty-five minutes three times a week performed better in psychological tests than people who merely did stretching and toning exercises.[9]

How to exercise

For those of us who have no gardening to do or messages to deliver on the other side of a mountain, the only opportunity for incidental exercise we get may be when we stroll over to the office water cooler from time to time. Some of us even glide to the water cooler on our swivel chairs. We tell ourselves there is 'no time' to take exercise, but it's strange how easy it can be to fit in several hours' worth of TV viewing after work instead. You can actually incorporate regular exercise into your busy life quite easily, as long as you have the willpower. Experts recommend half an hour to one hour of reasonably strenuous exercise most days of the week in order to get the benefits.

Walk briskly

The best kind of exercise works on the whole body simultaneously, including the muscle groups, skeletal system, circulatory system, nervous system, respiratory system and immune system. Brisk walking for half an hour meets all these criteria, and because it is a weight-bearing exercise it strengthens the bones and so helps to prevent osteoporosis.

Brisk walking can be done anywhere, at any time – try walking to work instead of taking the bus. Brisk walking is probably better for you than jogging, which can cause knee injuries and has also been found to reduce immune cell levels.[10] The best longevity-promoting exercise mimics the kind of movements our bodies make naturally; weightlifting, for example, will not improve your health as much as walking or swimming will, although it will tone your muscles.

Take aerobic exercise

The true benefits of exercise will only occur when the exercise is aerobic. The deeper breathing brought about by aerobic exercise helps oxygen and nutrients get to the places where they are needed and boosts heart function.

Types of aerobic exercise include brisk walking, swimming,

dancing, climbing uphill, riding, roller blading, rebounding, tennis, football and martial arts – anything that makes you out of breath. Belly dancing, although not especially aerobic, is good for stiff backs and the pelvic area, and seems to create extra amounts of endorphins. Yoga is an excellent form of exercise that acts like aerobic exercise by oxygenating the tissues through deep breathing. Yoga can benefit internal organs and improve the flow of lymph and blood flow, and there are yoga exercises for specific complaints such as constipation and flatulence.

Don't overdo it

Do not be tempted to over-exercise. It increases levels of ageing free radicals and suppresses the immune system. This is why professional athletes tend to have short careers and often have to retire as a result of health problems, especially immune-system-related illness. Too much exercise increases levels of the ageing stress hormone cortisol. One of many studies in this area showed that runners who run long distances and have low-fat diets have suppressed immune systems and raised levels of cortisol and inflammatory prostaglandins.[11] For the best results, combine regular, moderate exercise with a diet based on wholefoods and the right kind of fats.

Take one step at a time

There is no need to totally overhaul your life in order to take in a major exercise programme. If you are not in the habit of getting any exercise at all, start with just a few minutes a day and work gradually upwards – you will soon find you don't feel right without your daily bit of exercise and that you want more and more.

You could begin by walking or cycling to places you need to get to that are near enough, or even walking to the supermarket and carrying some moderately heavy bags back instead of driving. If you don't want to move away from the TV or stereo, you can do step aerobics on a step at home in front of the TV, or buy a rebounder and jump around for ten minutes to music.

IN SUMMARY

Exercise

- Exercise helps you to feel younger, look better and live longer.

- A healthy diet works best in tandem with regular aerobic exercise.

- Exercise can negate the effects of bad habits such as smoking to a certain extent.

- Try to take half an hour to an hour of aerobic exercise most days of the week; a little is better than none at all.

chapter

20

Don't worry yourself to death

•

A sad soul can kill you quicker, far quicker, than a germ.

JOHN STEINBECK, American novelist, 1902–1968

LONG-LIVED POPULATIONS LIVE IN THE MOMENT, not regretting yesterday or worrying about tomorrow. Their daily preoccupations are to do with growing their crops, socialising and getting around the mountains and fields where they live. They exist in extended families, where problems are divided and people work towards common goals, such as getting the wine harvest in. We, on the other hand, have to worry about relationships, mortgages and jobs. There are, however, many ways in which you can reduce the stress in your life, and plenty of enjoyable anti-stress habits you can borrow from long-lived people like the Hunzakut, Bama and others.

What is stress?

No one is exempt from stress. Too much work, too little work, traffic jams, no spouse, a spouse, moving house, divorce and death – the reasons to be stressed are unrelenting, with a new one usually popping up its ugly head as soon as the last has been dealt with. This is why people who plan to give up smoking 'as soon as the stressful situations stop' are on a losing streak. We have limited control over the number of potentially stressful situations that we will have to encounter during our lives. We *are*, however, able to choose how we respond to such situations, whether it be like Buddha or like Mad Max.

Mechanisms for coping with stress were useful in the past when we were, say, fleeing from a herd of stampeding elephants; they are less useful today when we are, for instance, trapped behind our desk by a belligerent boss. When you are stressed, your body switches into 'fight-or-flight mode', ready to run away from the source of danger. Your heart beats faster, your breath quickens and your blood pressure rises. Your body makes stress hormones such as adrenalin and cortisol, glucose is released into the bloodstream and your cholesterol levels rise. Potassium and phosphorus are excreted, which makes your body more acid, and free radicals are formed. Your digestion, libido and immune response are put on hold while energy is diverted elsewhere.

Every one of these mechanisms also just happens to cause accelerated ageing and diseases of ageing. Thousands of years ago, when we just had the odd fight-or-flight situation, this was not a problem, but today many people are chronically stressed. Stress devastates the immune system; researchers estimate that chronic stress contributes to up to 80 per cent of all major illnesses, including cancer, heart disease and back problems.[1]

The first physical signs of stress include fatigue, irritability, inability to concentrate, insomnia and drinking too much. If you find that, mysteriously, you always seem to get ill as soon as you have a day off or go on holiday, you can be fairly sure that you are suffering from stress. Stress hormones suppress the symptoms of illness, so as soon as the cause of the stress is removed, the symptoms surface.

People who are resistant to stress have been found to live longer and enjoy better health than others. Jeanne Calment, the Frenchwoman who lived for a record 122 years, was known for being unflappable and immune to stress. The New England Centenarian Study found that people who live long lives tend to have 'stress-resistant personalities'.[2] A person's attitude can even affect the progress of cancer. When Dr David Spiegel of Stanford University studied women with meta-stasised breast cancer, he found that those who joined support groups lived twice as long as those who did not, and that the experimental group also had half as much pain as the control group.[3]

It is believed that one reason why women tend to live longer than men is that they have better mechanisms for dealing with stress, such as the ability to talk about their problems. In Campodimele, the men actually often outlive the women; this may be due to their stress-free lifestyles and the ability of Mediterranean men in general to release their feelings.

Reducing your stress levels

All of the following activities and attitudes have been found to reduce stress levels and promote health. If you suffer from stress, try to incorporate some or all of them into your daily routine.

Laugh for ten minutes each day

The health craze for laughter – otherwise known as 'inner jogging' – was born in the US in the 1960s, when *Saturday Review* editor Norman Cousins made an extraordinary recovery from illness. He was diagnosed with a painful autoimmune disease called ankylosing spondylitis, from which he was told he had a 1 in 500 chance of recovering. He was sent to hospital, where he was given thirty-eight painkillers daily as well as sleeping pills and codeine.

Worried about the effects of this medication along with the abysmal food he was given, Cousins decided that hospitals were no place for sick people and had himself discharged. Aware of the negative effects of stress on health, he reasoned that the opposite must also be true, and set about inventing his own laughter cure.

Every day Cousins watched Marx Brothers films from his bed and had his nurse read amusing books to him. He soon found that if he had a good ten-minute belly laugh each day, he was able to have two hours of pain-free sleep. Within a relatively short space of time, Cousins was well enough to return to his job full-time.[4] He was ridiculed for his methods at the time, but his findings have since been backed up by several scientific studies.[5]

Plan, don't worry

By undertaking to cure himself, Norman Cousins showed how effective it can be to take an active role in your own health rather than taking the doctor's verdict for granted. For one thing a doctor may be wrong, and for another, you have the power to affect the outcome. Dr Max Gerson, pioneer of the Gerson Therapy for cancer patients, once stated that more people diagnosed with cancer die of panic than from the disease. Feeling out of control or helpless is a source of stress, and it can produce toxins and exacerbate an illness.

If a stressful situation arises and there is nothing you can do about it, then at least you can alter the way you feel about it. There is nothing wrong with making plans, but worrying is pointless. When the future does come, it will be the present, and it will not be how you imagined it.

Love someone – or get a dog

Marriage can be for better *or* worse health. One recent study showed that married people live longer and enjoy better health than single people (if you aren't married, read on as there is another side to the coin). The study, conducted by Warwick University, showed that married people, especially men, live up to three years longer, and that living together does not have the same effect.[6]

Reasons given for the longevity-promoting effects of marriage included a sense of security and having someone to talk to about your problems, which men often find difficult to do outside of marriage. Another reason could be sexual healing: according to neuropsychologist Dr David Weeks, sex three times a week between long-term partners can make women in particular look up to ten years younger, partly because it produces growth hormone in women.[7] Sex three times a week outside a stable relationship, however, may age single women, perhaps because it brings about insecurity.

It is the quality of the marriage that counts, however, since being in a bad relationship has been found to shorten lifespan. Scientists at Ohio State University found that couples who were nasty and sarcastic towards each other during fights had weakened immune systems, with women being more susceptible than men.

Another disadvantage of being married, according to British Nutrition Foundation dietician Sarah Schenker, is that marriage makes women fatter, as they tend to take on their husband's bad eating habits, such as eating crisps.[8] Male partners can disrupt women's sleep, especially if they snore. The Warwick study also found that cancer rates are highest amongst divorcees, with the cost of divorce lawyers (at £150 per hour) contributing to the stress caused.[9]

The people described earlier come from societies that have supportive extended family networks, and they do not have unrealistic expectations about marriage. What studies on marriage show is not that you must get married, but that you can improve your health by surrounding yourself with a supportive network, if not through a partner, then through friends, family, a counselling group or therapy. Pets also prolong life and are known to keep blood pressure down – University of Warwick researchers found that getting a dog also makes you three times more likely to meet people of either sex.

Give more than you receive

Selfish people die younger than helpful people, according to a recent study. University of Michigan researchers followed a group of older people for five years and found that those who were helpful to others were 60 per cent more likely to outlive those who weren't. Strangely, being on the receiving end made no difference; researchers concluded that the benefits of being in relationships are more to do with the giving than the receiving (in theory, this means that you can give away your expensive anti-ageing face cream and still get the benefits). Scientists have also found that being hostile is an even better predictor of heart disease than unhealthy living habits such as drinking and smoking.[10] The people discussed in Part I live in communities and remember each other's needs and have time to devote to each other.

Meditate yourself younger

According to studies, people who practice transcendental meditation (TM) have an incredible 55 per cent less cancer and 80 per cent less heart disease than non-meditators.[11] Meditation also improves eyesight, hearing and blood pressure. According to one study, those who meditate for five years or more measure five years younger biologically than those who don't.[12] During meditation, the body goes into a profound state of restfulness similar to that experienced in the deepest sleep; this state of being is the exact opposite of fight or flight, and could be called the 'rest-and-repair' state. Both the Okinawans and the Hunzakuts achieve serenity with regular meditation sessions.

Meditation consists simply of putting the attention on the breath, focusing on nothing – or *now* – and bringing the mind back to nothing whenever it starts to wander or thoughts crowd in. Meditation takes commitment, which is where its deep and long-lasting benefits lie. For a quick fix, lie face up on the bed or floor, imagine a peaceful scene such as a tropical beach, then breathe in deeply through your nose and out through your mouth for five or ten minutes. At the end you should feel refreshed and rested but alert.

Get enough sleep

Edward L Schneider, of the Leonard Davis School of Gerontology, UCLA, says 'To age successfully, you must get a good night's sleep.' Deep, good-quality sleep is particularly important for hormone production, immune function, digestive function and energy. A study by the American Cancer

Society in the 1950s showed that those sleeping for less than four hours a night or for more than nine or ten hours had the highest mortality, while those sleeping for eight hours had the lowest mortality. Deep sleep is encouraged by a good diet, regular exercise and an avoidance of stress. The long-lived populations that have been described tend to get eight hours of quality sleep every night.

Get spiritual

The people featured in this book have strong spiritual beliefs, whatever their religion. Being religious may or may not give you eternal life, but it is likely to lengthen it: most doctors will tell you that personal prayer, meditation or other spiritual practices can enhance medical treatment.

One study of 3,900 Israelis over sixteen years revealed that religious Israelis were only half as likely to die during that time period as their non-religious counterparts, even taking into consideration factors such as age and financial circumstances.[13] Another large epidemiological study in Maryland, US showed that church attenders were around half as likely to die from heart disease or suicide as non-churchgoers, and 74 per cent less likely to die from liver cirrhosis.[14] This seems to be not just because attending church is a social activity but also because spiritual beliefs give people a sense of meaning and a feeling that they are being looked after.

IN SUMMARY

Being stress free

Stress causes illness and premature ageing. Ways to reduce stress levels in your life include:

- Laughing for ten minutes or more each day.

- Feeling in control of your life and health.

- Enjoying harmonious relationships.

- Planning rather than worrying.

- Being generous.

- Meditating.

- Sleeping eight hours a night – but not much more than that.

- Having spiritual beliefs.

III

Putting it all together

The final section of this book summarises the information in the earlier parts and includes some further useful tips on healthy eating and other factors that help to increase longevity.

The secrets of living long in summary

W HAT ARE THE SECRETS OF LIVING LONG and staying young, in a nutshell? The fifteen 'secrets' of the long-lived populations described in this book are encapsulated below, along with a suggestion for an ideal daily intake of different types of food that will help you to stay young.

If you follow the outlined suggestions, the likely benefits to you should include:

- Prolonged youth

- Long life

- Plenty of energy

- Youthful looks

- Slender figure

- Positive outlook

- Higher IQ

- Happy bowels

- Trouble-free menstruation

- Clear skin

- Shiny hair

- Robust immune system

- Healthy offspring

- Less likelihood of serious chronic illnesses such as cancer, heart disease, stroke, diabetes and Alzheimer's disease

The fifteen 'secrets'

Here's a summary of the fifteen 'secrets' I've outlined in Part II.

1. Eat exactly what you need

Aim to eat no more than 2,200 calories daily, of food that is rich in nutrients. This means having a diet that is based on fruits, vegetables and whole grains, and including essential fatty acids from oily fish, nuts and seeds, and fresh cold-pressed nut and seed oils.

2. Eat a variety of fruits and vegetables

Eat five to ten servings daily of fresh fruits and vegetables, and try to eat foods of several different colours at each meal so as to get the full spectrum of anti-ageing antioxidants working together to quench ageing free radicals. Red wine is rich in potent antioxidants, but limit it to one glass daily for women and two glasses for men.

3. More raw foods

Eat raw foods for their high nutrient value and enzyme content. Try to eat as large a proportion of your food raw as possible, in the form of salads, raw vegetables and fruits.

4. Less meat and more vegetable protein

Cut down on your meat and dairy intake, as these foods are high in damaging saturated fats. Eat vegetable protein instead, in the form of beans and pulses, and nuts and seeds.

5. Keep your blood vessels young

Avoid premature death from cardiovascular disease by keeping cholesterol and homocysteine levels low, ensuring you get enough vitamin C, and avoiding high blood pressure by not getting stressed and eating healthily.

6. Eat the right fats

Make sure you eat the right types of fat – essential fats – which are essential for good health and the proper functioning of your body. Avoid saturated fats and, worse, hydrogenated fats, which cause disease. This means regularly including oily fish, nuts and seeds in your diet, and avoiding animal proteins and processed foods.

7. Eat whole grains

Eat whole grains such as brown rice and wholewheat flour, and avoid refined carbohydrates such as white rice and white flour. Whole grains contain valuable nutrients and keep your blood sugar levels stable, whereas refined carbohydrates drain the body of nutrients and cause dangerous fluctuations in blood glucose and insulin levels.

8. Mind your stools

Look after your digestion, as you cannot achieve good health from a nutritious diet unless your body can absorb and assimilate the nutrients properly.

9. Detox, don't botox

Detoxify regularly with methods such as fasting and sweating out toxins, and try to avoid overloading your body with toxins from pollution and junk foods. Drink eight glasses of water daily to flush toxins through your system and keep your body hydrated.

10. Be immune to ageing

Boost your immune system with a healthy diet, plenty of exercise and relaxation techniques; a strong immune system is essential if you want to avoid all kinds of illnesses from colds to cancer.

11. Eat food for thought

Keep your brain young with a healthy diet based on fruits and vegetables, whole grains and essential fats.

12. Eat organic and avoid 'Frankenfoods'

Eat organic food when possible so as to get the maximum amount of nutrients possible from your food.

13. Supplement your diet

Take vitamin and mineral supplements so as to insure against illness caused by nutrient deficiency; much of the fruit and vegetable produce sold in Western supermarkets is low in nutrients as a result of being grown in poor-quality soil.

14. Exercise, exercise, exercise

Get plenty of regular exercise and fresh air; aim for half an hour to an hour daily of brisk aerobic exercise. A healthy diet works hand in hand with an exercise programme to keep you fit and youthful.

15. Don't worry yourself to death

Avoid age-promoting stress with methods such as laughing, meditating and developing loving relationships.

The ideal daily diet

Your ideal daily diet should be as similar as possible to the diets of the people that were described in Part I. It should incorporate the following each day:

FRUITS AND VEGETABLES

Five to ten servings of fruits and vegetables – preferably one to two servings of fruits and the rest vegetables, mainly raw or lightly steamed.

COMPLEX CARBOHYDRATES

Four servings of whole grains such as brown rice, whole wheat, oats, corn, quinoa, hemp and/or millet.

PROTEIN

Three servings of vegetable protein from tofu, quinoa, lentils, or other beans or pulses; occasional small amount of organic cheese (preferably sheep's or goat's milk), yoghurt, a free-range organic egg or lean meat.

ESSENTIAL FATS

A handful of nuts and seeds *or* 1 tablespoon cold-pressed nut and seed oils *or* 1 heaped tablespoon ground seeds *or* fish oil supplements (daily) *or* oily fish (twice weekly).

Note: one serving is equivalent to 100 g (4 oz) grains, one large carrot or one slice of bread.

DRINKS

You should also aim to drink eight glasses of water daily, plus one or two cups of green tea.

chapter

22

More on ageing substances

●

ERE IS SOME SUPPLEMENTARY INFORMATION on the ageing 'foods' and substances you should avoid. All of these are notably absent from the diets and lifestyles of the people discussed in Part I. I've also included an example of the type of daily diet that you should avoid.

Fast foods

These speed up the ageing process with artery-hardening fats, salt and free radicals, even if they save you time in the short term. An example of the ideal ageing meal might be a hamburger or fried chicken in a white bap, accompanied by chips and a fizzy drink or milk shake, followed by a sugary snack or pie.

Cigarettes

Smoking a packet of twenty cigarettes a day is believed to add around eight years or more to your biological age. If you stop, you can undo much of the damage; in five years you can reverse most of the accelerated ageing that has taken place. If you do smoke, you have a one in two chance of dying an unpleasant, premature death as a result.

Excess alcohol

A small amount of wine, especially red wine, is good for you, and as mentioned previously it is drunk in moderation by many long-lived people. However, more than one (for women) or two (for men) drinks daily, especially of spirits, will signifi-cantly speed up the ageing process – alcoholics nearly always look much older than they really are.

According to Dr Gene-Jack Wang of Brookhaven National Laboratory in New York, 'the brain of a thirty-year-old alcoholic looks like the brain of a fifty-year-old'. Limit your drinking to moderate amounts of wine, preferably red, drunk with a meal. The liver has incredible powers of rejuvenation, so don't ever feel that it is too late to change your bad drinking habits.

Pharmaceutical drugs

Drugs are harmful, which is why they must be kept out of reach of children, and they should not be regarded as cures because they merely suppress symptoms. In doing so, they can inhibit the body's efforts to heal itself and maintain its normal, balanced condition. They cannot be metabolised easily, and the body expends valuable energy in trying to process them. They create ageing free radicals and cause side-effects, many of which are harmful to the liver.

Even a drug as seemingly innocuous as aspirin, which is touted as helping to prevent heart disease, may cause damage to the stomach and gut lining, leading to digestive problems and hence to various illnesses. Long-term use of non-steroidal anti-inflammatory drugs (NSAIDs) such as aspirin and ibupro-fen causes 20,000 deaths in the United States each year.

If your doctor has prescribed drugs, make sure you discuss it with them and only take them if you feel there is no alterna-tive – many drugs are unnecessary and are given as placebos.

Sugar

Sugar is probably the most degenerated food there is. Commercial sugar is a bleached product that is almost a pure carbon, and forms carbonic acid in the body. Carbonic acid is toxic to tissues, and must be neutralised with any spare mineral reserves the body has, so that they become increasingly depleted the more sugar is eaten.

Sugar stresses the adrenal glands, causes acne, and promotes yeast and fungal overgrowth in the body. It is high in calories and is converted to saturated fat in the body. It can increase your risk of developing conditions such as heart disease, varicose veins, kidney disorders, arthritis, diabetes, obesity, migraines, and high blood pressure. It also feeds cancer cells, and particularly increases the risk of getting breast cancer or cancer of the colon. The average North American eats fifty-seven kilograms of sugar annually in the form of biscuits, cakes, sweets, soft drinks, ketchup and spreads.

Sugary foods seem very pleasant because they are addictive. However, like all addictions, a sugar addiction can be reversed by simply avoiding any sugar for a few days. Try eating a piece of ripe fruit or a handful of dried fruits if you really want a sugary snack. If you like chocolate, choose dark semi-sweet chocolate, which is made from 70 per cent cocoa solids and raw cane sugar, and does not contain hydrogenated vegetable oil or vegetable fat.

Caffeine

The link between coffee drinking and degenerative disease is becoming increasingly clear. According to studies, drinking coffee may increase the risk of diabetes by impairing insulin function, and it contributes to high blood pressure by raising blood homocysteine and triglyceride levels.[1] Caffeine also halves the amount of nutrients absorbed with a meal.

Caffeine, like sugar, is addictive, and it is possible to get rid of the addiction by avoiding coffee for a few days. If you really cannot give up your coffee, try to get your intake down to one cup a day, and drink it away from a meal so that you still get your nutrients. After a while, you will notice that you feel quite jittery and unpleasant if you have more than this. Tea is better than coffee, as it contains slightly less caffeine and also includes antioxidants. Green tea has anti-ageing properties and the least caffeine content, and is drunk by some of the long-lived populations discussed in this book.

Salt

Those who are not used to cooking without salt often say that salt gives food 'taste'; others think it just makes food taste of salt. Salt increases blood pressure and therefore raises the risk of heart disease. The use of salt is strictly prohibited in cancer cures such as the Gerson Therapy as it disrupts the sodium–potassium balance that is so crucial to healthy cell function.

Salt causes fluid retention, as it must be kept in solution in the body, and so can cause swelling of parts of the body such as the ankles. You need some salt, as it is used in nerve transmission and keeping the balance of water in the body, but you can get it from natural foods and do not have to add it to your cooking.

Heavy metals and plastics

Canned food, tap water, mercury amalgam fillings and contaminated meat are all sources of toxic heavy metals that can accumulate in the body and cause degenerative disease. Canned tuna fish, for example, contains high levels of mercury, while aluminium foil, pans and antacids may all cause a build-up of aluminium in the body, which has been linked to illnesses such as Alzheimer's disease. Children's teeth braces made with nickel are associated with above-normal levels of appendicitis, for unknown reasons. The most common heavy metals found in human tissue at potentially harmful levels are cadmium, mercury, lead, aluminium, arsenic and nickel.

Plastics used in cling film and plastic packaging contain hormone-disruptive chemicals that are linked with conditions such as infertility and hormone-related cancers. Try to avoid wrapping food in cling film at home – you can put it in a bowl with a plate on top instead, or cover it in such a way that the cling film does not touch the food. Hard plastic, such as that used in plastic boxes and bags, is preferable to the soft plastic that is used in cling film and many supermarket wrappings.

A daily diet that you should avoid

This is the reverse of the ideal diet (*see page 256*). It strongly resembles the SAD (Standard American Diet), a diet that is comparable to other diets in the West. It is low in nutrients and high in 'empty calorie' foods such as saturated fats and sugar, which are fattening but do not feed the body. Combine this diet with a high-stress, low-exercise lifestyle and you have the ultimate formula for ill health and accelerated ageing.

Coffee and fizzy drinks One or more cups of coffee and/or sweet fizzy drinks.

Sweets One or more servings of chocolate, cakes, sweets or biscuits.

Alcohol Over two glasses of alcohol daily, especially spirits.

Altered fats One or more servings of foods containing hydrogenated fats such as ready meals, packaged cakes and biscuits, or foods fried in vegetable oil, such as chips,

Saturated fats One or more servings of meat, especially red meat, and full-fat dairy products.

Fast foods One or more meals from fast-food outlets.

Refined carbohydrates Two and above servings of white bread, white rice, biscuits, cakes or pastry.

Tips for using the 'secrets'

•

IT IS ONE THING TO BUY A BOOK ABOUT HEALTH FOOD, and another to actually do what it tells you to do. If you want to benefit from the invaluable information available in nutrition books today, you have to get into the habit of eating healthy food *almost always*, rather than just now and again. The odd deviation won't kill you, but eating the wrong way all the time might.

It's amazing how many of us do not eat healthily, but think we do. This is hardly surprising – healthy eating isn't taught at home or in schools, and much of the information put out is confusing and conflicting. Corn flakes with milk for breakfast, and chicken sandwiches on semi-brown bread with a tiny bit of iceberg lettuce, washed down with orange juice or coffee and a vitamin pill for lunch, is not healthy eating, even if it seems as though it is. If you eat this way and wonder why you still get spots, unshiftable love handles, premenstrual syndrome and headaches (to name but a few), you will be amazed by how much better you look and feel when you eat *really* healthily.

Enjoy cooking and eating your food

You don't have to think about the concepts behind healthy eating if you don't want to. You can just cook it, enjoy it, and feel the energy and health miraculously coursing into your grateful body, just as the excess pounds fall off. Eating should not be punishing or sacrificial. You are making a commitment, however, and this will mean putting in the work that a change of habit requires.

You will have to make time to go to the supermarket or health-food shop and to prepare the food. You will probably soon find, however, that not only is this extra effort well worth it, but that the effort itself – choosing and preparing food – becomes a rewarding part of your day. As you begin to explore new ingredients, impress your friends with your new cooking skills, feel and look better, and are complimented on how well you look to the point where it bores you, you won't look back.

When using the principles in this book, make things easy for yourself by discovering which foods you like best and are easiest to shop for and prepare, then use them regularly. There is no point in having soya every day for a week and tomatoes the next week, then never having either of them again. People living in long-lived communities eat their health foods on a regular basis, in moderate quantities, so that they get the cumulative benefits over a lifetime. If you particularly like green tea and buckwheat, make them some of your staples and using them will become a habit.

When planning meals, shop adventurously, remembering that there are dozens of different kinds of fruits, vegetables, whole grains, fish and other healthy foods around. Avoid the central aisles of the supermarket, which is where the cakes and biscuits tend to be, and spend more time in the vegetable section and exploring different kinds of food which you like at the health-food shop. Invent your own recipes using the principles of healthy eating, and try using oriental and Mediterranean cookery books to expand on your repertoire as well as the recipes in this book.

Each of us is unique, and everyone responds to different types of food in their own way. Experiment to find out which foods suit your digestive system and give you energy, and which do not. When you start eating healthily, your body becomes more able to discern what it does and does not thrive on, and you should become able to spot the signs. You may feel lethargic or flatulent after eating bread, for example, which you might not have noticed before if you were feeling like this all the time.

One step at a time

If you hate the idea of missing out on doughnuts and crisps, set a goal of eating healthily for one month only, and focus on what you would like to improve about your health. At the end of the four weeks, you will probably feel so much better that you will want to continue eating this way. When you eat clean, healthy food, the body detoxifies and the taste buds become more appreciative, so you may lose your taste for doughnuts and crisps anyway.

Like cigarettes, these 'foods' are cleverly manufactured to be addictive, and after a brief period of withdrawal they often lose their appeal. In fact, research has shown that once people get away from their established tastes, they start enjoying health-giving foods. One of my favourite foods used to be pizza, but I remember vividly having my first pizza after several months of strict healthy eating, and I was amazed to find that it tasted like cardboard and rubber.

Whatever you do, don't 'diet'. Make sure you always satisfy your appetite and that you make your food as delicious as possible. Keep healthy snacks such as fruits or nuts around to eat between meals if you get hungry. At meal times, if you are having a salad don't make it from watery, tasteless iceberg lettuce and tomato, because you will just be wishing you were having something else. Throw in lightly roasted sesame seeds, olives, herbs and anything else you can find to make it interesting.

Occasional indiscretions

The benefits of lightly steamed vegetables or poached fish will be severely compromised if you top them off with a bowlful of ice cream, even if it is eaten surreptitiously with your head inside the freezer. However, if you do stray into the arena of unhealthy eating from time to time, try to adapt sensibly. If you find you've just had three pints of beer and a kebab before you even knew what you were doing, don't then think you have ruined everything and eat hamburgers and pizza for the rest of the week in an orgy of guilty masochism. Just forget what happened and get back on track by continuing as before.

If you love red meat or white bread and would rather not live a long time if it means going without them, have them from time to time. Just change the ratios around so that you have more of the vegetables and less of the unhealthy foods, and try not to indulge too often. I find that men generally seem to like meat more than women do, so if you are a health-conscious woman cooking for a man who just wants his meat (or vice versa), you can deceive him by making a vegetable-based dish flavoured with small amounts of meat (that's how the people described in Part I eat theirs). If you love a warm white baguette or focaccia bread, try to eat it as a special treat only and stick to whole grains at other times.

Eating out

If you are going to a restaurant or don't feel like cooking and want to get a takeaway, try to stick to the principles of healthy eating as far as possible. If you can, persuade the people you are meeting to go to a Japanese restaurant or one that does vegetarian food, and there is bound to be an option on the menu that suits you. If you have to go somewhere where there is nothing that you want on the menu, order the best option and ask if you can have an extra helping of steamed green vegetables or a salad on the side. Most restaurants keep food in the kitchen that isn't on the menu and will be happy to oblige. You can then concentrate on the vegetables and leave some of the main dish.

If you are eating dinner at someone's house, whoever is cooking may well show their hospitality and their fondness for you by trying to give you severe indigestion. Your plate is heaped high, you are urged to eat a second or third helping, an enormous slice of treacle tart is placed firmly in front of you. If this happens only on rare occasions, just enjoy it. Otherwise you must forget everything your mother taught you and leave something on your plate – or simply ask for small portions (you can always say tactfully that you are on a diet!).

The office lunch

It can be hard to find anything to eat other than sandwiches around the office, so if you are dedicated enough you might have to make your own lunch and bring it in. I remember starting a new job and cautiously lifting the lid off my Tupperware box containing brown rice, soy sauce, garlic and seaweed with broccoli and beans, slightly embarrassed by the garlicky smell that wafted out. I was surprised when two or three people stopped on their way past my desk to ask what I was eating. One of them was inspired to start doing the same herself at lunchtime, and the other placed an order with me to make lunch for her too, which I did every day from then on.

Stocking up

Stock up on a range of foods that you can incorporate into your healthy eating plan so that they are always ready to be cooked at home. Rather than putting them at the back of the cupboard where you might forget them, place them in glass jars on a shelf where they will look attractive and remind you of their presence. Do not leave them in open bags, which will decrease spoilage times and may attract health-conscious insects and rodents.

Items you can stock up on

- Extra-virgin olive oil.

- Organic whole grains, beans and pulses (brown rice, brown rice cakes, whole-grain flour, polenta, porridge oats, lentils, a variety of beans).

- Nuts and seeds for snacks (unsalted, uncooked nuts, sunflower seeds, sesame seeds and pumpkin seeds).

- Dried fruits for snacks (apricots, dates, figs).

- Oriental noodles (such as Somen and Udon noodles, available in health-food shops and oriental supermarkets).

- Kombu seaweed for making Dashi (available in packages from health-food shops and oriental supermarkets).

- Bonito flakes for making Dashi (sachets of dried fish flakes available in oriental supermarkets).

- Miso soup (available in sachets from health-food shops and supermarkets).

- Tofu.

- Garlic.

- Growing herbs.

- A selection of dried herbs.

- Green tea.

- Herb tea.

Finally, *enjoy* doing the Live Longer Diet. Try to make food you like and engage in exercise and relaxation practices that are within your reach, so that you can stick with it. Set your sights on the here and now and appreciate the immediate benefits of the 'secrets' – after all, even more important than living longer is feeling good *today*.

References

Introduction

1. *European Journal of Human Genetics*, 31 October, 2002; 10:682–688
2. Ernst Krebs Jr., 1974 speech at the 2nd Annual Cancer Convention, Ambassador Hotel, LA, California (from Phillip Day, *Cancer: Why We're Still Dying to Know the Truth*, Credence Publications, UK, 1999
3. www.drmcdougall.com/Newsletter/jan–feb.99.1.html
4. Dr Michael Colgan, quoted from www.miraclehealth.com/goodnews.3.htm
5. British Heart Foundation website
6. Cancer Research UK 1998 statistics, Cancer Research UK website
7. The Cancer Cure Foundation website, www.cancure.org
8. Day, P., *Cancer: Why We're Still Dying to Know the Truth*, Credence Publications, UK, 1999
9. Report by Chief Medical Officer, Professor Liam Donaldson, reproduced in report by MP David Davis, 2001

CHAPTER 1

1. Suzuki, M., MD, Willcox, B., MD, Willcox, C., PhD., *The Okinawa Way*, Penguin Books Ltd, UK, 2001
2. Weindruch, R., and Sohal, R., 1997 'Caloric intake and aging' *New England Journal of Medicine* 337(14):986–994
3. Suzuki, M., Akisaka, M. and Inayama, S., 1993 'Medicobiological studies on centenarians in Okinawa, measuring plasma lipid peroxide, proline, and plasma and intracellular tocopherol'. In Beregi, E., Gergely, I.A. and Rajczi, K. eds., *Recent Advances in Aging Science* Bologna:Monduzzi
4. *Nutrition and Cancer*, 1994, 21;2:113–131
5. Dr Hidemi Todoriki, Japan Public Health Center Database – note 45, Chapter 2, *The Okinawa Way*
6. *Journal of Nutrition*, March 1995, 125;3:606S–611S

7. *American Journal of Clinical Nutrition*, Dec 1998, 68;6:1453S–1416S
8. Rice, M., 'Soy consumption and bone mineral density in older Japanese American women in King County, Washington'. The Nikkei Bone Density Study. University of Washington 1999, PhD dissertation; Alekel, D.L., St. Germain, A., Peterson C.T. et al., 'Isoflavone-rich soy protein isolate attenuates bone loss in the lumbar spine of perimenopausal women'. *American Journal of Clinical Nutrition*, 2000, 72:844–52
9. Study conducted by Dr Lon White at the Pacific Health Research Institute
10. National Institute for Longevity in Tokyo study reported in the *Daily Mail*, 27 November, 2000
11. Study by Oxford University/Cancer Research UK, secretariat Professor Valerie Beral, *British Journal of Cancer*, Nov 12, 2002
12. Gao, Y.T., McLaughlin, J.K., Blot, W.J. et al., 'Reduced risk of esophageal cancer associated with green tea consumption'. *Journal of the National Cancer Institute* 1994, 85:855–58; Katiyar, S.K. and Mukhtar, H., 'Tea in chemoprevention of cancer: epidemiologic and experimental studies'. *International Journal of Oncology* 1996, 8:221–38
13. As reported by Jean Carper, *Stop Ageing Now!* HarperCollins, 1995 (p201)
14. Wallace, R.K., Dillbeck, M., Jacobe, E. and Harrington, B., 'The effects of transcendental meditation and TM-Sidhi program on the aging process'. *International Journal of Neuroscience*, 1982 16:53–58
15. Willcox, D.C., Todoriki, H., Sakihara, S., Willcox, B.J., Naka, K. and Ariizumi, M., 2000 'Minority aging in Japan: subjective well-being of older Okinawans in cross-cultural context' (unpublished)

CHAPTER 2

1. Karagiannis, S., Karagiannis, N., Grigoriadis, E. and Telonis, M., 1994 *Comparison of morbidity and causes of death between the province of Rhodes and the rest of Greece, during the decade 1981–1990*. 14th Panhellenic Gastroenterology Conference. Athens 16–20 Nov, 1994
2. From Burton Goldberg, *Heart Disease, Stroke and High Blood Pressure*, Future Medicine Publishing, Inc., USA p200
3. *Experimental Gerontology* 32:149, 1997
4. Jean Carper, *Stop Ageing Now!* HarperCollins, 1995 (p159)
5. *Epidemiology*, 18 Feb, 1998
6. Dr Sinatra's views reported by Burton Goldberg, *Heart Disease, Stroke & High Blood Pressure*, Future Medicine Publishing, Inc, USA, 1998 (p182)

CHAPTER 3

1. *Alimentazione, Nutrizione, Invecchiamento; 2a Campodimele Conference, Obiettivo Longevita*, Edizioni L. Pozzi, 1995
2. *Alimentazione, Nutrizione, Invecchiamento; 2a Campodimele Conference, Obiettivo Longevita*, Edizioni L. Pozzi, 1995

CHAPTER 4

1. As reported in an article by Sir Robert McCarrison, 1925
2. Hoffman, Dr J. F., *Hunza – Secrets of the World's Healthiest and Oldest Living People*, 1960
3. Mellon Lecture, Pittsburgh, USA, 1922, Sir Robert McCarrison
4. *American Heart Journal*, Dec 1964
5. Taylor, R., *Hunza Health Secrets*, Keats Publishing Inc, USA, 1964
6. Leaf, Dr A., *National Geographic*, Jan 1973
7. Rodale, J. I., *The Healthy Hunzas*
8. Krebs, E., 1974, speech at the Second Annual Cancer Convention, LA. In Day P., *Cancer: Why We're Still Dying to Know the Truth*, Credence Publications, UK, 1999

CHAPTER 5

1. *China Geriatrics Magazine*, 1982 (11) (2)
2. Ze Yang; Systematic Research and Analysis of the Factors Associated with Longevity in Bama Population, 1981; Zhi-Chien Ho, MD., 'A study of longevity protein requirements of individuals 90–112 years old in southern China'. *Journal of Applied Nutrition*, 1982 (34) (1)
3. Ze Yang; Systematic Research and Analysis of the Factors Associated with Longevity in Bama Population, 1981
4. *European Journal of Human Genetics* 31 Oct, 2002; 10:682–688
5. Zhang Yan, et al., 1994
6. Ze Yang; Systematic Research and Analysis of the Factors Associated with Longevity in Bama Population, 1981
7. Study from Cornell University, *Journal of Agriculture and Food Chemistry*
8. Ze Yang; Systematic Research and Analysis of the Factors Associated with Longevity in Bama Population, 1981
9. Zhi-Chien Ho, MD., 'A study of longevity protein requirements of individuals 90–112 years old in southern China'. *Journal of Applied Nutrition*, 1982 (34) (1)
10. Health Longevity Survey in China, Peking University and China National Research Centre on Ageing

CHAPTER 6

1. Walford, R.L. and Walford, L., *The Anti-Aging Plan*, Four Walls Eight Windows, NY, 1995
2. Walford, R.L. and Walford, L., *The Anti-Aging Plan*, Four Walls Eight Windows, NY, 1995
3. Self, *New England Journal of Medicine*, Nov 1995
4. Ko Ho Duncan, et al., *American Journal of Clinical Nutrition 37*, 1983:763
5. As reported in *The Week*, issue 360 1/6/02

CHAPTER 7

1. Carper, J., *Stop Ageing Now!* HarperCollins, USA, 1995
2. In this study Gladys Block, PhD., of the University of California, Berkeley, analysed data from 170 studies from 17 countries
3. Optimum Nutrition Newsletter *100% Health*, Issue 3

CHAPTER 8

1. Quote from Leslie and Susannah Kenton, *Raw Energy*, Guild Publishing, 1984 (p89)
2. Quote from Leslie and Susannah Kenton, *Raw Energy*, Guild Publishing, 1984 (p89)

CHAPTER 9

1. Krohn, P., 1972. 'Rapid growth, short life'. *Journal of the American Medical Association*, 1959, 171:461
2. Professor Nick Day, *Cambridge University and European Prospective Study into Cancer*, Thorogood, 1994
3. Dickerson, J.W.T. et al., 'Disease patterns in individuals with different eating patterns'. *Journal of the Royal Society of Health,*1985, vol 105, p191–4
4. Colin Campbell, Dr T., 'Some snippets of information from the China Project'.
5. Colin Campbell, Dr T., MS, PhD, *Nutrition Advocate* vol 1, 1995 No 6, Dec
6. Reddy, B. and Wynder, E., 'Large bowel carcinogenesis: fecal constituents of populations with diverse incidence of colon cancer'. *Journal of the National Cancer Institute*, 1973, 50:1437

7. Obituary Column, p C-11, *Riverside Herald*, 14 March, 1982

8. Kolata, G., 'Major study links animal fats to cancer of colon'. *New York Times*, 13 December, 1990

9. Lagerquist, R. and McGregor, T., *North American Diet*; University of Massachusetts Medical School, *Journal of the National Cancer Institute*,1998

10. Sandhu, M.S. et al., 'Systematic review of the prospective cohort studies on meat consumption and colorectal cancer risk: a meta-analytical approach'. *Cancer Epidemiology, Biomarkers and Prevention*, 2001, 10:439–446

11. *Science News*, 23 April, 1994

12. Norrish, A.E., Ferguson, L.R., Knize, M.G. et al., 'Heterocyclicamine content of cooked meat and prostate cancer'. *Journal of the National Cancer Institute* 91, 1999 (23):2038–44; Commoner, B., Vithayathil, A.J., Dolara, P. et al., 'Formation of mutagens in beef and beef extract during cooking'. *Science*, 1978, 201:913–16

13. Dosch, H.M., 'Interview with Hans-Michael Dosch – an update of the Ig-G-mediated cow's milk and insulin-dependent diabetes connection, part 2'. *The Immunological Review*, vol 2:3 (Spring 1994)

14. Walker, A, 'The human requirement of calcium: should low intakes be supplemented?' *American Journal of Clinical Nutrition*, 1972, 25:518

CHAPTER 10

1. From New Century Nutrition
   <http://www.newcenturynutrition.com/NCN/articles/spelling_trouble.html>.

2. Willcox, B., MD, Willcox, C., PhD, and Suzuki, M., MD, *The Okinawa Way*, Michael Joseph, 2001

3. Rath, M., and Pauling, L., 'Hypothesis: lipoprotein(a) is a surrogate for ascorbate'. *Proceedings of the National Academy of Sciences of the USA* 87:16 (Aug 1990), 6204–6207

4. 'Reducing hypertension: is diet better than drugs?' *Alternative & Complementary Therapies* 3:1 (Feb 1997)

5. Goldstein, I.B., et al., 'Home relaxation techniques for essential hypertension'. *Psychosomatic Medicine* 46:5 (Sept/Oct 1984), 398–414; The Joint National Committee on Detection, Evaluation, and Treatment of High Blood Pressure, 'The 1988 Report of the Joint National Committee of the American Medical Association', *Archives of Internal Medicine* 148 9 (1988), 1023–1038

6. Gordon, L., 'Exercise and salt restriction may be enough for mildly high blood pressure'. *Medical Tribune* 8 (21 December, 1995)

7. Fortmann, S.P. et al., 'The association of blood pressure and dietary alcohol: differences by age, sex and estrogen use'. *American Journal of Epidemiology*, 118:4 (October 1983), 497–507; Gruchow, H.W. et al., 'Alcohol, nutrient intake, and hypertension in U.S. adults'. *Journal of the American Medical Association*, 253:11 (March 1985), 1567–1570

8. Lang, T. et al., 'Relation between coffee drinking and blood pressure: analysis of 6,321 subjects in the Paris region'. *American Journal of Cardiology* 52:10 (December 1983), 1238–1242

9. From Burton Goldberg *Heart Disease, Stroke, and High Blood Pressure*, Future Medicine Publishing Inc, 1998 (p175–6); He, J., et al., 'Oats and buckwheat intakes and cardiovascular disease risk factors in an ethnic minority of China'. *American Journal of Clinical Nutrition* 61 (1995), 366–372

10. Stephens, N. et al., 'Randomised controlled trial of vitamin E in patients with coronary disease: Cambridge Heart Antioxidant Study (CHAOS)'. *Lancet*, (23 March, 1996) 347; *Hypertension* 22:3 (September 1993), 371–379

11. Meneely, G.R. and Battarbee, H.D., 'High sodium-low potassium environment and hypertension'. *American Journal of Cardiology* 38:6 (November 1976), 768–785

12. Foushee, D.B., Ruffin, J. and Banerjee U., 'Garlic as a natural agent for the treatment of hypertension: a preliminary report'. *Cytobios* 34 (1982), 135–136, 145–152

13. *The Nutrition Practitioner*, 3.1, March 2001

14. From Burton Goldberg *Heart Disease, Stroke, and High Blood Pressure*, Future Medicine Publishing Inc, 1998 (p36)

CHAPTER 11

1. Erasmus, U., *Fats that Heal, Fats that Kill,* Alive Books, 1986, 1993

2. *New England Journal of Medicine* vol 323 no 7, 1990, 437–445; Willet, 1994

3. Budwig, J., *Flax Oil as a True Aid against Arthritis, Heart Infarction, Cancer and Other Diseases*, Canada, Apple Publishing, 1994

4. Simopoulos, A., *American Journal of Clinical Nutrition* vol 54, 1991, 438–463

CHAPTER 12

1. Salmeron, J., Manson, J.E., Stampfer, M.J., Colditz, G.A., Wing, A.L. and Willet, W.C., 'Dietary fiber, glycemic load and risk of non-insulin-dependent diabetes mellitus in women'. *Journal of the*

American Medical Association 1997; 277:472–477; Salmeron, J., Ascherio, E.B., Rimm, G.A. et al., 'Dietary fiber, glycemic load and risk of NIDDM in men'. *Diabetes Care*, 1997; 20:545–550

2. 'Findings from Bristol Royal Hospital for Sick Children'. *Daily Mail* article by Beezy Marsh, 28 Sept, 2002
3. Carper, J., *Stop Ageing Now!*, HarperCollins, 1995 (p284)
4. Garg, A., Grundy, S.M. and Unger, R.H, 'Comparison of effects of high and low carbohydrate diets on plasma lipoproteins and insulin sensitivity in patients with mild NIDDM'. *Diabetes*, 1992; 41; 1278–1285; Mensink, R.P., de Groot, M.J.M., van den Broeke, L.T., Severijnen-Nobels, A.P., Demacker, P.N.M. and Katan , M.B., 'Effects on monounsaturated fatty acids v complex carbohydrate on serum lipoproteins and apoproteins in healthy men and women'. *Metabolism* 1989; 38:172–178
5. Smith, M.A. et al., 'Advanced Maillard reaction end products are associated with Alzheimer disease pathology'. *Proceedings of the National Academy of Sciences USA* 1994; 91:5710–5714; Vitek, M.P. et al., 'Advance glycation end products contribute to amyloidosis in Alzheimer's disease'. *Proceedings of the National Academy of Sciences USA* 1994; 91:4766–4770
6. Hankinson, S.E., Willett, W.C., Colditz, G.A. et al., 1998. 'Circulating concentrations of insulin-like growth factor-I and risk of breast cancer'. *Lancet* 351:1393-96; Giovannucci, E., 1995. 'Insulin and colon cancer'. *Cancer Causes Control* 6 (2):164-79; Chan, J., Stampfer, M., Giovannucci, E., 1998. 'Plasma insulin-like growth factor I and prostate cancer risk: a prospective study'. *Science* 279 (5350):563–66.
7. Al-Abed, Y. et al. 'Inhibition of advanced glycation endproduct formation by acetaldehyde: role in the cardioprotective effect of ethanol'. *Proceedings of the National Academy of Sciences USA* 1999; 96:2385-90
8. *Lancet*, 18 May, 1996; 347:1351–1356

Chapter 13

1. Burkitt, D., 'Dietary Fiber and Disease'. *Journal of the American Medical Association*, 1974, 229:1068

Chapter 14

1. Reported by Ian Belcher, 'The enema within'. *Guardian*, UK, 9 March, 2002

2. Reported by Ian Belcher, 'The enema within'. *Guardian*, UK, 9 March, 2002

3. Sokol Green, N., *Poisoning Our Children*, Noble Press, 1991

CHAPTER 15

1. Vanderhaeghe, L.R. and Bouic, P.J.D., PhD, *The Immune System Cure*, Cico Books, London, 2001

2. Kijak, E., Foust, G. and Steinman, R., 'Relationship of blood sugar level and leukocytic phagocytosis'. *Southern California State Dental Association Journal* 32, No. 8, September 1964

3. Keicolt-Glaser, J.K. et al., 'Modulation of cellular immunity in medical students'. *Journal of Behavioural Medicine*, vol 9:5 (1986)

4. McCraty, R., Prodeedings of the Tenth International Montreux Congress on Stress, Montreux, 1999

5. 'The effect of light, moderate and severe bicycle exercise'. *International Journal of Sports Medicine*, vol 14 (5)

CHAPTER 16

1. Suzuki, M. et al., *The Okinawa Way*, 2001

2. Reynolds, B.A. and Weiss, S., 'Central nervous system growth and differentiation factors: clinical horizons – truth or dare?' *Current Opinions in Biotechnology* 4(4) 1993:734–38

3. Agostoni, C. et al., 'Docosahexaenoic acid status and developmental quotient of healthy term infants'. *Lancet*, Vol 346,2 Sept, 1995, 638

4. Burgess, J.R. et al., 'Long-chain polyunsaturated fatty acids in children with attention-deficit hyperactivity disorder'. *American Journal of Clinical Nutrition*, Vol 71 (suppl), Jan 2000, 327S–30S; Stordy, B., 'Dark adaptation, motor skills, docosahexaenoic acid, and dyslexia'. *American Journal of Clinical Nutrition*, vol 71 (suppl) January 2000, 323S–26S

5. Stoll, A.E. et al., 'Omega-3 fatty acids in bipolar disorder: a preliminary double-blind placebo controlled trial'. *Archives of General Psychiatry*, 1999; 56:407–412

6. Hibbeln, J.R. et al., 'A replication study of violent and nonviolent subjects: cerebrospinal fluid metabolites of serotonin and dopamine are predicted by plasma essential fatty acids'. *Biological Psychiatry*, Vol 44 No 4, 15 Aug, 1998, 243–249

7. Sano, M. et al., 'A controlled trial of slegiline, alpha-tocopherol, or both as treatment for Alzheimer's disease'. *New England Journal of Medicine*, 24 April, 1997; 336:1216

8. Study by E. B. Healton and colleagues, Columbia-Presbyterian Medical Center
9. Godrey, P.S.A., Reynolds, E.H. et al., 'Enhancement of recovery from psychiatric illness by methylfolate'. *Lancet* vol 336, 1990, 392–395
10. As reported by Dr Jay Lombard and Carl Germano, *The Brain Wellness Plan*, Kensington Publishing Corp, USA, 1997 (p199)
11. Leslie and Susannah Kenton, *Raw Energy*, 1984
12. Reported in Patrick Holford, *The Optimum Nutrition Bible*, Piatkus Ltd, 1997 (p147)
13. Vitek, M.P., Bhattacharya, K., Glendening, J.M. et al., 'Advanced glycation end products contribute to amyloidosis in Alzheimer's disease', *Proceedings of the National Academy of Sciences USA*, 1994; 91:4766–4770
14. Dr Eleanor Maguire, *Proceedings of the National Academy of Sciences*, 2000

Chapter 17

1. Robbins, J., *Diet for a New America*, H.J. Kramer, USA, 1987
2. Vidal, J., 'M&S calls on other stores to ban pesticides'. *Guardian*, 8 August, 2002
3. 26 March, 1981, *New England Journal of Medicine*
4. Child cancer rates 'Increasing', BBC news online, 18 December, 2001; *Lancet*, Sept 2002. Maastricht Ageing Society, Netherlands
5. Report by Anita Manning, 'Biotechnology ready to grow but critics would shuck it all, even the less-fatty fries'. *USA Today*,14 Dec, 2000
6. 'Genetically modified crops and food'. Friends of the Earth briefing, note 10 (available online)
7. 'Genetically modified crops and food'. Friends of the Earth briefing, note 29 (available online); 'Genetically modified crops and food'. Friends of the Earth briefing (available online)
8. 'The Fear of Food'. *Newsweek*, 27 January, 2003
9. 'Genetically modified crops and food'. Friends of the Earth briefing
10. Brown, J. and Brown, A.P., 'Gene transfer between canola and related weed species'. *Annals of Applied Biology*, Vol 129 (1996) 513–522
11. 'Genetically modified crops and food'. Friends of the Earth briefing (note 27)

Chapter 18

1. Carper, J., *Stop Ageing Now!* HarperCollins USA, 1995 (p51)

2. *British Medical Journal*, 1997 314:634–8

3. Carper, J., *Stop Ageing Now!* (p60)

4. Klipstein-Grobusch, K., Geleijnse, J.M., den Greeijen, J.H. et al., 'Dietary antioxidants and risk of myocardial infarction in the elderly: the Rotterdam Study'. *American Journal of Clinical Nutrition* 1999:69:261–266; Carper, J., *Stop Ageing Now!* (p61)

5. Diplock, 1994

6. Carper, J., *Stop Ageing Now!* (p44); Knekt, P. et al., 'Serum vitamin E level and risk of female cancers'. *International Journal of Epidemiology* 17 (1988) 281–286

7. Stampfer et al., *New England Journal of Medicine* June 1993

8. Carper, J., *Stop Ageing Now!* (p119)

9. Clark, L.C. et al., 'Effect of selenium supplementation for cancer prevention with carcinoma of the skin: a randomised controlled trial'. *Journal of the American Medical Association* 1996, 276:1957–1963

10. Study by Professor Harold Foster, University of Victoria, British Columbia, (as reported in Lorna R. Vanderhaeghe and Patrick J.D. Bouic, PhD, *The Immune System Cure*, Cico Books, UK, 2001)

11. Suadicani, P., Hein, H.O. and Gyntelberg, F., 'Serum selenium concentratin and risk of ischaemic heart disease in a prospective cohort study of 3000 males'. *Atherosclerosis* 1992; 96:33–42; Carper, J., *Stop Ageing Now!* (p119)

12. Carper, J., *Stop Ageing Now!* (p97)

13. As reported by Burton Goldberg, *Heart Disease, Stroke and High Blood Pressure*, Future Medicine Publishing, USA, 1998 (p118)

14. Folkers, Dr K., *Clinical Investigator* (as reported in Lorna R. Vanderhaeghe and Patrick J. D. Bouic, PhD, *The Immune System Cure*, Cico Books, UK, 2001)

15. Lockwood et al. (as reported in Lorna R. Vanderhaeghe and Patrick J. D. Bouic, PhD, *The Immune System Cure*, Cico Books, UK, 2001)

16. Carper, J., *Stop Ageing Now!* (p144)

17. Maydani et al., 1995

18. As reported in Lorna R. Vanderhaeghe and Patrick J. D. Bouic, PhD, *The Immune System Cure*, Cico Books, UK, 2001

19. Rayssiguier, Y., 'Magnesium and aging. I. Experimental data: importance of oxidative damage'. *Magnesium Research*, 1996

20. Wood, D.A. et al., 'Adipose tissue and platelet fatty acids and coronary heart disease in Scottish men'. *Lancet* 2:8395 (July 1984) 117–121

21. Dr Richard Anderson, Beltsville Human Nutrition Research Centre, Maryland: 180 patients with Type II diabetes were given 200 mcg chromium piccolinate daily and their blood glucose levels were

lowered, comparable or even better than most medication used for Type II diabetes.
22. Carper, J., *Stop Ageing Now!* (p75)

CHAPTER 19

1. Stanford study reported in *Newsweek*, 20 January, 2002
2. Thune, I., Brenn, T. et al., 'Physical activity and the risk of breast cancer'. *New England Journal of Medicine* 1997; 336:1269–1275; Tang, R., Wang, J.Y., Lo, S.K. and Hsieh, L.L., 'Physical activity, water intake and risk of colorectal cancer in Taiwan: a hospital-based case-control study'. *International Journal of Cancer* 1999; 82:484–489
3. *Journal of the American Medical Association* October 2002
4. Clapp, J.F., 'Exercise and fetal health'. *Journal of Developmental Physiology* 1991;15:14; Frankel, T., 'Walking may protect hips'. *Prevention Magazine*, 8 February, 1990
5. Pierog, J.E., RN, MS, NC, 'Recipe for longevity', Healthlinks.net newsletter
6. Wei, M., Gibbons, L.W., Mitchell, T.L. et al., 'The association between cardiorespiratory fitness and impaired fasting glucose and type 2 diabetes mellitus in men'. *Annual of Internal Medicine* 1999; 130:89–96
7. Leveille, S.G., Guralnik, J.M. et al., 'Aging successfully until death in old age: opportunities for increasing active life expectancy'. *American Journal of Epidemiology* 1999; 149:654–664
8. Lennox, S.S., Bedell, F.R. and Stone A.A., 'The effect of exercise on normal mood'. *Journal of Psychosomatic Research*, 1990;34(6):629–636; Braverman, E.R., 'Sports and exercise: nutritional augmentation and health benefits'. *Journal of Orthomolecular Medicine*, 1991;6:191–200.
9. Kramer, A.F., Hahn, S., Cohen, N.J. et al., 'Ageing, fitness and neurocognitive function'. *Nature* 1999; 400:418–19
10. Shore, S., Shinkai, S. et al., 'Immune responses to training: how critical is training volume?' *Journal of Sports Medicine and Physical Fitness*, 1999; 39:1–11
11. Presentation by J.T. Venkatramen, 4th International Society for Exercise and Immunology Symposium, May 1999

CHAPTER 20

1. Phyllis, A., Balch, James, C.N.C. and Balch, F. MD, *Prescription for Nutritional Healing*, Avery Books, USA, 2000 (p647)
2. Perls, T.T. and Silver, M.H., *Living to 100*, Basic Books, USA, 1999

3. Spiegel, D., Bloom, J.R. and Gottheil, E., 'Effects of psychosocial treatment on survival of patients with metastatic breast cancer', 1989

4. Cousins, N., *Anatomy of an Illness as Perceived by the Patient*, W.W. Norton & Co Inc, New York, 1979; Oswald, A. with Gardner, J., 'Is it money or marriage that keeps people alive?' 15 August, 2002 (report at www.oswald.co.uk)

5. Mook, B., 'Love and laughter: two things to help successful aging'; Silver Linings website

6. Oswald with Gardner, 'Is it money or marriage that keeps people alive?' 15 August, 2002 (report at www.oswald.co.uk)

7. Dr David Weeks, *Secrets of the Superyoung*

8. As reported by Andrea Thompson, 'Does marriage make you healthier?' *Glamour,* November 2002

9. Oswald with Gardner, 'Is it money or marriage that keeps people alive?' 15 August, 2002 (report at www.oswald.co.uk); as reported by Andrea Thompson, 'Does marriage make you healthier?' *Glamour,* November 2002

10. *Health Psychology*, November 2002

11. *Psychosomatic Medicine* 49 (1987): 493–507; Wallace, R.K., Dillbeck, M., Jacobe, E. and Harrington, B., 'The effects of transcendental meditation and TM-Sidhi program on the aging process'. *International Journal of Neuroscience* 16 (1982), 53–58

12. Wallace, R.K. et al., *International Journal of Neuroscience* 16 (1982), 53–58

13. Study by Jeremy Clark, 1996, *Chance News*, 1997

14. Comstock and Partridge, 1972

CHAPTER 22

1. Kiejzers et al., *Diabetes Care*, 2002; Thong et al., *Diabetes*, 2002; Grubben et al., *American Journal of Clinical Nutrition*, 2001; 71:480–4

Resources

Recommended Reading

Leon Chaitow, *Thorson's Principles of Fasting*, Thorsons/HarperCollins, UK, 1996

Phillip Day, *Cancer – Why We're Still Dying to Know the Truth*, Credence Publications, UK, 1999

Udo Erasmus, *Fats that Heal, Fats that Kill*, Alive Books, Canada, 1986

Charlotte Gerson and Morton Walker, DPM, *The Gerson Therapy*, Kensington Publishing Corp, NY, USA, 2001

Patrick Holford, *The Optimum Nutrition Bible*, Piatkus Publishers Ltd, UK, 1997

Gudrun Jonsson, *Gut Reaction*, Random House, 2000

Leslie and Susannah Kenton, *Raw Energy – Eat Your Way to Radiant Health*, Guild Publishing, London, UK, 1984

Elizabeth Lipski, MS, CCN, *Digestive Wellness*, Keats Publishing, USA, 1996

Jean A. Oswald, *Yours for Health – the Life and Times of Herbert M. Shelton*, Franklin Books, USA, 1989

John Robbins, *Diet for a New America*, H.J. Kramer, USA, 1987

Maria Wilhelmi-Buchinger, *Fasting: The Buchinger Method*, The C.W. Daniel Company Ltd, UK, 1984

Useful Addresses

The British College of Nutrition and Health
79 Compayne Gardens,
London NW6 3RW,
UK
Tel: +44 (0) 207 372 5740
Fax: +44 (0) 207 372 5789
www.bcnh.co.uk

Buchinger Fasting Clinics
Forstweg 39,
D31812 Bad Pyrmont,
Germany.
Tel: (00) (49) 811 660
www.buchinger.de

The Dove Clinic
(A clinic for integrative medicine including vitamin B17 treatment)
Tel: +44 (0) 207 486 5588
www.doveclinic.com

The Gerson Institute
PO Box 430, Bonita,
California 91908-0430,
USA
Tel: (001) 619 685 5353
www.gerson.org

GM crops
www.genewatch.org
Friends of the Earth GM crop/organic food campaign:
%20info@foe.co.uk

Mother Hemp Ltd.
(Hemp products suppliers)
Tilton Barns,
Firle, Lewes
East Sussex BN8 6LL,
UK
Tel: +44 (0) 1323 811 909
www.motherhemp.com

*The Herbology and Optimal Nutrition Education and Research
Institute*
46 10th Avenue
Boston 7530
South Africa
Tel: +27 082 626 0969

Nature Care College of Natural Therapies and Life Studies
79 Lithgow Street
St Leonards NSW 2065
Australia
Tel: +61 2 9438 3333

New Zealand Nutrition Foundation
C/- Private Bag 25 905
St Heliers
Auckland
New Zealand
Tel: +64 9 575 3419

Index

and nutritional supplements 225, 227, 228–9
and refined carbohydrates 174, 260
and salt 262
and stress 242
heavy metals 262
Helicobacter pylori 23
hemp 98–9, 108, 175–6
hemp oil 165
Hemp Pasta with Pesto 108
herbal tea 84
herbs 25, 40–1, 102
herring 20, 41
Hilton, James 72
Hippocrates 6, 179, 190
Hoffman, Jay F. 73
homocysteine 156–7
human immuno-deficiency virus (HIV) 200
Hunza, Pakistan 5, 72–92, 149, 165, 169, 175, 184, 190, 207, 208, 241, 247
  case study 86
  cooking methods 131
  diet 74–5, 76–7, 78–84
  dos and don'ts 87
  family structure 85–6
  farming practices 77–8, 217
  physical exercise 84–5, 235
  recipes 88–92
  traditional way of life 75–6, 85
Hunza water 84
hypertension 74, 76, 153–5, 236, 260
hypoglycaemia 170

ibuprofen 260
illnesses, top killers 8–12
immune system 198–206, 255
  boosting 201–5
  and stress 242
  stressors 203
insulin 170, 172, 203
insulin resistance 170, 171
intestinal flora 95, 181
iron 96, 143
Irons, V. E. 194–5
isoflavones 21

jasmine green tea 24
Jerome, Jerome K. 235
Jesus Christ 190
Jonsson, Gudrun 182

kamut 177
Kenton, Leslie 213

Kenton, Susannah 213
Kokkinos, Georgios 45–6
Kradjian, Robert 140
Krebs, Ernst, Jr 2–3, 79

lactase 142
lamb 42, 92
Lamb, Feta, and Pasta Stew 90–1
Lane, Arbuthnot 189
laughter 244
Leaf, Alexander 76–7
leaky gut syndrome 213
lemon balm 41
life expectancy 8–9
lifespan 1, 113
lipid peroxide 17
lipoproteins 151
Lipski, Elizabeth 196
livers 189
longevity 1–2
  desire for 118–19
  hotspots 4–5, 13–109
lung cancer 11, 24, 140, 228
lycopene 39, 59, 97

McCarrison, Robert 73, 74–5, 208
McCully, Kilmer S. 156
McDougall, John 9
mackerel 19–20, 41
magnesium 143, 155, 225, 232–3
maize 82, 99–100
malt drink 63
manganese 96
marjoram 40
marriage 245–6
meat 22–3, 42, 62, 82–3, 136–48, 254, 267
  consumption guidelines 147
  digestion 137–8
  and mental health 214
  processed 140
  as toxin 138–9
medicines 11, 12, 259–60
meditation 27, 247
Mediterranean diet 35, 37–44
mental gymnastics 103–4, 214–15
mental health 174, 207–15, 255
migraines 133, 213
milk 63, 83, 142–3
millet 82, 176
mint 40
Mitford, Nancy 168
Mixed Salad with Sesame Seeds and a Garlic and Olive Oil Dressing 70–1
Morgan, John 139